Fibreoptic Intubation

To Rachel, Billy and George, and to Mum and Dad, and Mike, for all their love

Fibreoptic Intubation

Dr Neil Hawkins MB BS, BSc, FRCA
Specialist Registrar Anaesthetist, Nottingham and
East Midlands School of Anaesthesia, Queens
Medical Centre, Nottingham NG7 2UH, UK

Dr Andrew Dyson MB ChB, FRCA
Consultant Anaesthetist, Kings Mill Centre for Health
Care Services, Sutton in Ashfield, Nottinghamshire
NG17 4JL, UK

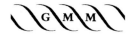

© 2000

Greenwich Medical Media Limited
137 Euston Road
London
NW1 2AA

ISBN 1 84110 060 9

First published 2000

A catalogue record for this book is available from the British Library.

Visit our website at:
www.greenwich-medical.co.uk

Distributed worldwide by Plymbridge Distributors Ltd.

Typeset by Phoenix Photosetting, Chatham, Kent
Printed by Grafos, Spain

Contents

Preface

This book is intended as an introduction to the fibreoptic laryngoscope and its use for intubation. An attempt has been made to cover all the main areas that a beginner should know about before embarking on the technique of fibreoptic intubation and a chapter on teaching the technique to others has also been included. At the end of the book are some useful facts and figures, addresses and a list of conditions known to be associated with difficult intubation.

A CD-ROM is included with the book, which contains video clips of important aspects of fibreoptic intubation.

The diagnosis and management of the difficult airway is a subject in its own right and cannot be covered adequately in a book of this size. Therefore, I have included in the bibliography some texts that examine this subject in more depth.

It is hoped that anaesthetists of all grades as well as related professionals, such as operating department practitioners and theatre nurses will benefit from this book.

Neil Hawkins

Foreword

It is very rare to be invited to write a foreword for a textbook, which has been written predominantly by a trainee. The reasons for using fibreoptic techniques are increasing and therefore, it follows that consultants and other anaesthetic staff should be well versed in the techniques. However, there is more to the subject than merely using a fibreoptic instrument. Thus, this book also looks at the broader aspects e.g. the physics of light transmission, construction and cleaning of instruments to mention but a few.

As most fibreoptic techniques are performed under sedation and local analgesia, it is important that the operator is able to acquire, demonstrate and teach both skills. The chapter on local analgesia is excellent and accompanied by equally excellent coloured pictures. They show the main nerves and their distribution thus assisting those wishing to obtain and develop these skills. As with any technique, or indeed any speciality, there are inevitably complications. Fibreoptic techniques are no exception and the possible complications and subsequent treatments are thoroughly discussed.

Experience is usually the result of successfully overcoming difficulties and treating complications. These lessons, which may have been painfully obtained, must be passed on to future generations so that they are neither lost nor repeated. Hence, there is a chapter included, which is designed to assist in terms of acquiring the necessary skills.

There is no doubt that the present generation of consultants and trainees will use fibreoptic techniques with increasing frequency. The teaching of such skills is therefore of paramount importance and has been thoroughly addressed. In addition, the author has added some useful appendices.

In the introduction, the authors' aim is to educate and promote safe practice in fibreoptic techniques. They have also stated that they would hope that other paramedical staff would also benefit. I believe that the authors have achieved their objective and that this textbook will be of great assistance to all those who seek to become competent in fibreoptic techniques. Finally, this book has been sponsored by Pentax and such an action must be applauded.

R S Vaughan
Consultant Anaesthetist
August 2000

Acknowledgements

Neil Hawkins gratefully acknowledges Pentax UK Ltd, Cook UK Ltd and Dr A. Norris for permission to use images and Pentax UK Ltd, Cook UK Ltd, Intavent UK Ltd and Laerdal UK Ltd for the use of equipment.

I would like to thank the following for their help, encouragement and support: Margaret, Louise, Adam, Gloria, Bailey, Simon Hardwick, Ken Kay, Dawn Churchill, Malcolm Brown, Robert Ibbotsen, Glynn Holmes, Donna Adams, Jill Hyatt, Brian Taylor, Andy Thomas, Nigel Kirkman, Professor Aitkenhead, Dr Ravi Mahajan, Dr Keith Girling, Dr Rob Scott, Dr Andrew Norris, Dr Mark Brown, Dr Caroline Bates, Dr Francis Spears, Mr Patrick Bradley, Liza Watson, Bob Plant, Geoff Langston, Andrew Smith, Sally Truman, Martin Clarke, Karen Gillard, Geoff Gilbert, Dave Hughes, Alan Minty, Paul Swann, Adrian Taylor, Geoff Nuttall, Gavin Smith, Nora Naughton, Richard Tebbits, the patients who gave permission to have their intubation recorded and all those who in some way made it easier for me to write this book.

Abbreviations and Glossary

Abbreviations

ASA	American Standards Association. It is a form of expression that indicates the light sensitivity (speed) of a photographic film.
BC	Before Christ
CD-ROM	Compact Disc Read Only Memory. These discs will hold approximately 650 megabytes of digital information, which can be downloaded from a computer hard drive via a compact disc writer.
cm	Centimetre
CPAP	Continuous Positive Airway Pressure
ETO	Ethylene Oxide
hr	Hour
kg	Kilogram
lb	Weight in pounds
litres/min	Litres per minute
LMA	Laryngeal Mask Airway
mg	Milligram
mg/kg	Milligrams per kilogram
MHz	Megahertz
ml	Millilitre
mm	millimetres
n =	Number equal to
UK	United Kingdom
X-rays	Radiographs
µg	Microgram
£	Pounds sterling
45°	45 degrees
°C	degrees centigrade
1:200,000	A dilution of 1 part in every 200,000
%	Percentage
~	Approximately
<	Less than

Word/Phrase — Definition

Word/Phrase	Definition
Antisialagogue	A drug that will inhibit the secretion of saliva e.g. the anticholinergic group of drugs such as glycopyrronium bromide and atropine.

Hanging-up	Anatomical obstruction of the easy passage of the endotracheal tube into the trachea e.g. when the tip of the endotracheal tube catches on part of the larynx.
Mallampati score	A system that attempts to identify the airway that will be difficult to intubate. It is based on the view obtained through the open mouth when the head and neck are in the neutral position and the tongue protruded. The system attempts to measure how obstructed the view is, based on which parts of the oral cavity and oro-pharynx are seen. The view is graded on a scale of 1 to 4.
Murphy's eye	The hole in the lateral wall of the tip of some types of endotracheal tube.
Railroading	The act of passing something over a guide e.g. the passing of the endotracheal tube over the insertion tube of a fibreoptic laryngoscope or a bougie.
Relative humidity	The ratio of the mass of water vapour in a given volume of air to the mass required to saturate that volume of air at the same temperature; expressed as a percentage.
Video capture card	A piece of computer hardware that will allow the computer to receive video signals. This enables video sequences to be saved to the computer hard drive.
Video capture unit	A processing unit that converts a video signal from a digital video camera into a signal that can then be recorded onto a video recorder.

Introduction

WHY DO YOU NEED TO KNOW ABOUT FIBREOPTIC INTUBATION?

The most common cause of mortality and serious morbidity due to anaesthesia is from airway problems. It is estimated that about one-third of all anaesthetic related deaths are due to a failure to intubate and ventilate. Not only are these cases disastrous for the patient and their family, the effect on the practitioner who failed to secure the airway must not be underestimated. Economically, there is often a high price to pay as well. If the patient survives and is brain damaged, they will require long term care. It is therefore incumbent on the anaesthetic fraternity to do as much as is possible to ensure that all anaesthetists are competent at managing the difficult airway. Failure to do so should be construed as a failure to discharge our duty to the best of our ability. During training one should not only teach the techniques used to manage the difficult airway, one should also emphasise that a rational approach is required when deciding which techniques would be safe to use in any given situation.

The flexible fibreoptic intubation laryngoscope gives the competent practitioner the unparalleled opportunity to secure almost any difficult airway encountered. Imagine a patient with a fixed and grossly flexed neck deformity, an inability to open the mouth, with one nostril blocked, a laryngeal tumour and who requires a procedure for which they need intubating. How would one feel facing this type of patient and how would one attempt an intubation? Intubation via the larynx can only be achieved safely by the practitioner skilled in fibreoptic intubation. If there is no one so skilled, then the patient may well be denied their operation. An awake tracheostomy may not always be possible if the neck is too flexed or if there is an anterior neck mass. Now imagine a morbidly obese drunken man in Accident and Emergency, with a Glasgow Coma Score of 5, with a history of having just eaten a large curry (after numerous pints of lager) and lying in the recovery position. It is probable that a supine rapid sequence induction is the way most practitioners would try to intubate the trachea of this patient, but it is feasible that the patient's body habitus and history could result in a failed intubation and the inhalation of the gastric contents. In the time it has taken to draw up the drugs for general anaesthesia, one can place an endotracheal tube into the trachea with a fibreoptic laryngoscope while the patient is still in the recovery position. The first example is fairly unlikely, but it illustrates the possibilities of the technique. The second example actually happened.

Flexible fibreoptic intubation is also a safe and relatively easy technique to learn. A study on patients with severe rheumatoid arthritis involving the neck showed that when compared with normal intubation, the fibreoptic group had significantly less trauma associated with intubation, and in the Northwestern Hospital in Canada, it was shown that 90% of the difficult or failed intubations were easy when performed fibreoptically. Why then would it appear that the number of anaesthetists proficient in the use of such a minimally traumatic and life-saving device is quite small? In 1992, a survey in the North of England showed that only 28% of consultants were deemed proficient in the technique and only one of 29 departments with teaching responsibilities actually had a formal training programme for fibreoptic intubation. These are such small numbers, despite 93% of the departments having a fibreoptic laryngoscope available. Many papers published on this subject comment on the reasons why this may be so. It is possible that in the early years, cost of the instrument and a lack of knowledge of the intricacies of the technique may have been prohibitive, and that later on the vicious circle of 'no one trained' therefore no one to learn from' was to blame. Practitioners who attempted the technique soon became discouraged by their failures and gave up. Another cause for the slow uptake among UK (see glossary) anaesthetists could be that fibreoptic intubation may have been used as a technique of last resort, when all other attempts at intubation had failed. This is not the best time to implement this technique; the airway is usually bloodied and the anaesthetist is tired, fed up and stressed. Attempts to fibreoptically intubate a patient at this stage can prove difficult and may fail, especially under general anaesthesia. This will just affirm to the practitioner that fibreoptic intubation is not such a great technique after all.

There are some recommendations about the use of the fibreoptic laryngoscope. In an editorial written in 1991, Dr Ralph Vaughan, Vice-President of The Royal College of Anaesthetists and former President of The Difficult Airway Society, recommended that all Anaesthetic departments should have a fibreoptic laryngoscope available and that training programmes be introduced in every department. As Dr Vaughan says, if fibreoptic intubation is the technique of choice for difficult intubations, then all anaesthetists should know how to perform it. In the 1996/97 *Report of the National Confidential Enquiry into Perioperative Deaths*, it is recommended that awake fibreoptic intubation should be considered among the options in the management of the obstructed airway, and that several individuals within a department should ensure that their competence with this technique is maintained. It also states that a 'fibreoptic laryngoscope should be readily available for use in all surgical hospitals'.

If we are to decrease the number of patients who are seriously handicapped or die from the result of failure to secure the airway, not only must we ensure that all the anaesthetists are competent at fibreoptic intubation, but also that the threshold to use the technique is lowered. When this happens, the difficult airway patient will be well counselled, well anaesthetised and safely intubated.

There are other advantages to having a fibreoptic laryngoscope. One can use it to assess upper airway pathology before arriving in theatre, to check the position of an endotracheal tube and see how far to draw it back, and to check the patency of a nostril before blindly passing a nasal tube. Fibreoptic laryngoscopes have even been used to position nasogastric tubes. The great advantage today is the advent of the portable fibreoptic laryngoscope, which can be used in theatre, in Accident and Emergency, in Intensive Care Units or just about anywhere a normal laryngoscope can be used.

2

The fibreoptic intubating laryngoscope (fibreoptic intubating scope, fibreoptic intubating bronchoscope, fibrescope or flexible laryngoscope)

HISTORY

PRINCIPLES OF FIBREOPTIC LIGHT TRANSMISSION

STRUCTURE OF THE FIBREOPTIC LARYNGOSCOPE

HANDLING OF THE INSTRUMENT

COST

The effect of the refraction, or bending of light, has been known since at least 300 BC when Euclid described it in his treatise *Catoptrics*. In 1611, Johannes Kepler described 'total internal reflection' of light (as if it had hit a mirror) in his monograph *Dioptrice*, and in 1621 Willebrord Snell van Roijen devised the laws pertaining to the refraction of light. In 1870 John Tyndall described how light could be contained within, and guided along, a stream of water. However, it was not until 1927 that a system was devised by John Logie Baird, the inventor of television, which enabled the transmission of optical images down thin glass bundles; unfortunately, the transmission of light down these early bundles was very poor. In the early 1950s Hopkins and Kapany did much of the developmental work on fibreoptics and named one of their systems the 'fiberscope', but it was 1956 before Lawrence Curtiss, at the University of Michigan, produced a glass fibre bundle capable of passing sufficient light to view objects well. This became the basis for the first flexible endoscope and it was suggested that it could be used to look into the stomach. Hirschowitz in 1957 reported the first use of the gastroscope.

The use of flexible fibreoptic instruments to help in airway management is a relatively recent event. In 1967, Dr P. Murphy was the first to use a fibreoptic instrument for the control of the airway when he performed a nasal intubation under general anaesthesia in a patient with advanced Still's disease. He used a choledochoscope to perform the intubation and even managed to take photographs through the scope. He then went on to use the choledochoscope for intubation with double lumen tubes.

The first fibreoptic bronchoscope was made in 1966, and in 1972 reports of the use of the fibreoptic bronchoscope for intubation were appearing in the academic literature. Initially, these scopes were of a large diameter and conventional fibreoptic intubation was not possible in young children. The first true fibreoptic laryngoscope became available in 1973 and over the years thinner scopes have been manufactured. By 1987, an ultrathin (2.7 mm, see glossary) fibreoptic laryngoscope had been designed and was being used to aid intubation in children with a difficult airway. Today, one can obtain scopes with an insertion tube as small as 2.4 mm.

Since the introduction of the fibreoptic laryngoscope many techniques and aids have been developed that cover almost every possible difficult airway problem.

PRINCIPLES OF FIBREOPTIC LIGHT TRANSMISSION

For a full understanding of how a fibreoptic laryngoscope works and why it is so important to handle, maintain and care for the instrument properly, knowledge of some basic physics is required.

Light travels at different velocities in different substances. The effect of each substance on light velocity is indicated by the 'refractive index' of the substance, which compares the velocity of the light through that substance with that through a vacuum. This difference in velocities has the effect of altering the direction of a light beam as it passes from one medium to another. If the light hits a glass–air interface at 90° (see glossary), it will pass straight through, but at any other angle, as the light passes from the glass to the air, its direction will be altered. As the angle of incidence of the light is increased from the perpendicular, the greater the bending of the light as it emerges from the glass into the air. Eventually, there will be a point where the light is reflected back inside the glass, almost as if it had rebounded off a mirror. This is called 'total internal reflection' and occurs at the 'critical angle' (Fig. 2.1). It becomes possible, therefore, to bounce light down the inside of a glass rod from one end to the other — and this is the basis of fibreoptics.

An important concept to appreciate is that the critical angle depends on the difference between the refractive indices of the two materials, e.g. the air and the glass. If similar glass rods are placed next to one another, there will be no bending of light and the light will carry on in its original direction (Fig. 2.2). If a liquid is placed outside the glass rod, it has a similar effect. It is therefore easy to understand how a fibreoptic endoscope can be ruined by allowing fluid to reach the fibreoptic bundles.

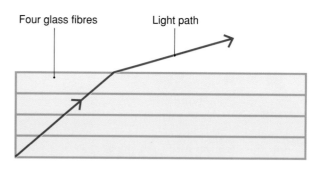

Fig. 2.2
Light will not reflect off the inside of a glass rod if several other similar rods are placed alongside it.

A fundamental problem when first designing the flexible fibreoptic endoscope, was how to make the glass rods thin enough to be flexible and how to bundle them together while keeping each fibre optically insulated from the others. Drawing out glass rods into thin fibres had been possible for a while, but it was Curtiss, working on the suggestion of Dr C. van Heel, who solved the internal reflection problem. In 1956, he managed to draw glass fibres of 0.0254 mm in diameter from a high refractive index glass rod coated with a layer of a low refractive index glass. This mimicked the effect of having a glass rod in air, so that many fibres could be bundled together with little or no loss of internal reflection, each fibre remaining optically insulated from the others. It was an elegant answer to a difficult problem (Fig. 2.3).

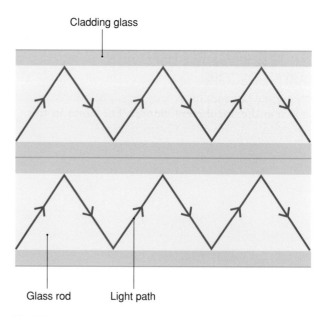

Fig. 2.3
Light can travel down the inside of two glass rods without interference.

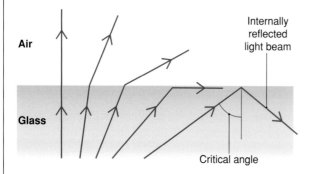

Fig. 2.1
Changing angle of refraction of a light beam when passing from one medium to another.

Another problem that had to be overcome was the means by which one could transmit not just light, but a coherent image down a fibreoptic bundle. This was achieved by arranging all the fibres in the viewing bundle of the instrument in a fixed position within the bundle. In other words, if a fibre starts at the tip of the instrument in the 12 o'clock position, it will emerge at the eyepiece end of the scope in the same position. This gives a picture at the eyepiece rather than a random array of light. This type of bundle is labelled as 'coherent'. A typical coherent, or viewing, bundle will have between 36,000 and 85,000 individual fibres, depending on the size of the instrument, each fibre being 6–10 μm in diameter. These fibres are arranged into small bundles, which are then placed together to form the viewing bundle (Fig. 2.4). It is the smaller bundles that can break when a fibreoptic scope is treated harshly, the outcome of which is the appearance of black dots in the viewed image.

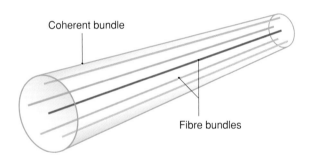

Fig. 2.4
Internal arrangement of fibres in the viewing (coherent) bundle.

A light-transmitting, or light bundle, only needs to pass a sufficient quantity of white light to illuminate the desired object, so the fibres can lie in any configuration. This is why the light bundle is known as the 'incoherent' bundle. The fibres in this type of bundle are ~10–15 μm in diameter.

STRUCTURE OF THE FIBREOPTIC LARYNGOSCOPE

Components

The fibreoptic laryngoscope consists of a few parts, which are all incorporated into a functional unit:

- Control body/handle
- Insertion tube/cord
- Umbilical/universal cord
- Light source

Control body/handle

The control body is used to hold and manipulate the instrument. It can be held in either hand, but one side usually feels the better. It has been suggested that it should be held in the left hand, but personally I find it easier to manipulate the scope and its controls using my dominant hand.

The control body is made up of several components:

- Body
- Eyepiece
- Control lever

Body
This is the part of the instrument that fits into the hand so that one can hold the instrument and rotate the insertion tube. Attached to the body is the control lever. It is also the part of the instrument that contains the viewing apparatus as well as the suction and injection ports (if the scope has a working channel, the smaller paediatric scopes are too narrow to accommodate one). Sometimes the injection port is separate from the suction button, while in other scopes the two are incorporated into the same port. There is also a suction nipple to which a suction unit can be connected. In a portable scope the light and its battery will also form part of the handle, but usually the umbilical (universal cord) is attached to the side (Figs 2.5 and 2.6).

Eyepiece
The eyepiece is the focusing element of the scope that can be adjusted to an individual's eyesight by turning the diopter or focusing control ring, which is situated at the top of the control body, just under the lens. It can be used to focus the scope on something before performing an intubation, so that a sharp image will be obtained when the endoscopy is performed. The 'depth of field', or depth over which things appear focused, is ~3–50 mm. If a video camera attachment is being used over the eyepiece, it is worth slightly de-focusing from the fully focused position as this will minimise the appearance of the ends of the fibre bundles that look like a lattice over the screen image. There is a triangular marker at the top of the endoscopic view, and this is to aid orientation (Fig. 2.7). There are also electrical contacts around the eyepiece for photography attachments.

Control lever
The control lever is near to the top of the control body. When the instrument is held in the neutral position, the control lever faces the chest of the

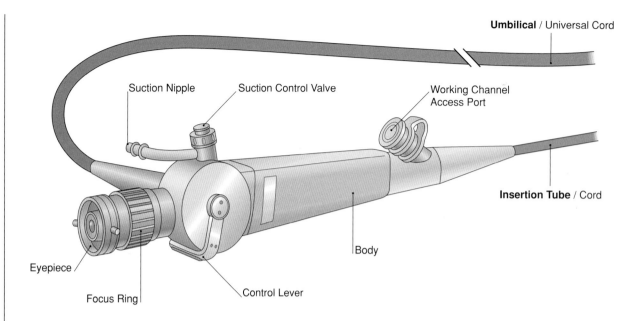

Fig. 2.5
Control body of a fibreoptic laryngoscope with the umbilical abutting on the side.

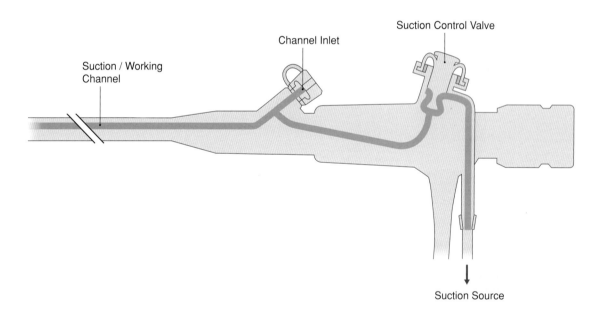

Fig. 2.6
Internal structure of the suction/working channel.

operator and it is best controlled with the thumb (Fig. 2.8). The lever controls two thin wires, which travel from it to the tip of the scope and activate the up and down movement of the last 2–3 cm (see glossary) of the insertion tube. The only thing to remember about the lever is that when it is depressed, the tip rises. The reverse happens when the lever is elevated. This can be confusing during the first few endoscopies when there is more to concentrate on than just the scope.

Insertion tube/cord

The insertion tube/cord is the 55–60 cm flexible fibrescopic element of the instrument that hangs from the handle and is inserted into the patient. It is longer than the equivalent bronchoscope, so that an uncut endotracheal tube can fit over the insertion tube and there still be enough length left to reach the mid-trachea before the tip of the endotracheal

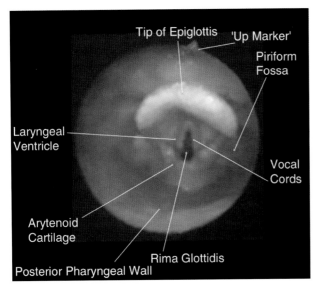

Fig. 2.7
Adult larynx through a fibreoptic laryngoscope. Note the 'up marker', which helps with scope orientation.

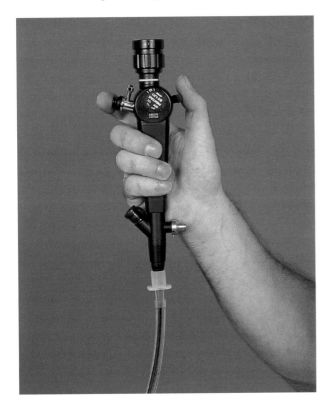

Fig. 2.8
Note the thumb on the control lever and the index finger controlling the suction valve. Also note how the endotracheal tube has been mounted over the tapered section of the control body.

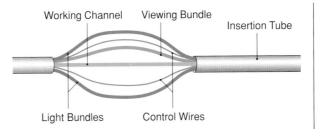

Fig. 2.9
Internal construction of the insertion tube of a fibreoptic laryngoscope.

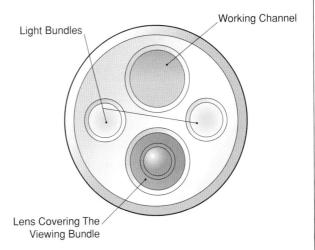

Fig. 2.10
Distal tip.

tube is next to the patient. Within it are the viewing (coherent) bundle, between one and three (though usually two) light bundles (incoherent), the two wires to control the tip of the instrument and usually a suction/working channel (Fig. 2.9).

All these components are encased in a thin, flexible, plastic polymer cover, which is constructed more strongly than on other endoscopes so that it can withstand the repeated railroading (see glossary) of an endotracheal tube. The terminal 2–3 cm is jointed, and as indicated, the lever on the handle controls its angulation at any time. At the very end of the insertion tube is a lens that focuses the image to be transmitted on to the end of the viewing fibreoptic bundle (Fig. 2.10). This light is then transmitted up the viewing bundle to the eyepiece, where the image is viewed. It will be found that the image quality is not as good in those scopes with a narrow insertion tube. This affects both subject illumination and image quality as both the viewing and the light bundles are smaller. Earlier scopes had only one light bundle that created a 'hot spot' on the image.

This part of the fibreoptic laryngoscope is extremely delicate and deserves respect. Damage here can result in a repair bill of thousands of pounds.

Umbilical/universal cord

The umbilical arises from the side of the control body. The light bundle, which the umbilical contains, transmits light from the light source to the scope and then down the insertion tube to illuminate the object to be viewed. The umbilical needs to be inserted into a light source and has a metal rod connector on its end for this purpose. There are also electrical wires within the umbilical that supply the photography contacts situated around the eyepiece.

Light source

Traditionally, this is a metal box sitting to the side of the instrument to which the umbilical attaches (Fig. 2.11). The source produces a cold, white light from a halogen, xenon or a newer metal halide lamp. Metal halide lamps are smaller and cheaper to buy and should last 300–400 hr (see glossary). Xenon lamps are expensive and last ~500 hr (see glossary). Some light boxes will contain all the circuitry necessary for flash photography, and some scope systems are made so that by the use of adapters the light source connector will fit any light source.

Portable scopes

Recently, fibreoptic laryngoscopes that do not need an umbilical have been introduced. Instead, a light

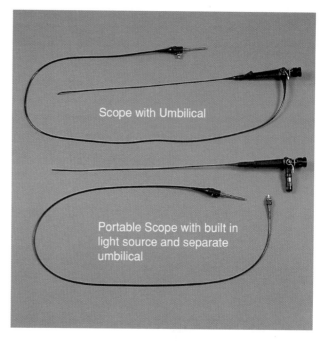

Fig. 2.12
Portable scope with battery light source attached, and a traditional scope (F1–10BS).

source is built into the control body of the laryngoscope. Power is supplied by a battery system contained within a small holder that is attached to the control body, which will normally give ~90 minutes of continuous use before it needs replacing. The great advantage of this type of scope comes from its portability. This portability is not a new idea, having been used as far back as 1973. However, if a conventional light source is preferred, an umbilical can be attached to the position where the battery holder screws onto the handle (Fig. 2.12).

Digital scopes

Digital flexible endoscopic systems are now being developed. A CCD chip is placed at the tip of the scope, which relays digitised information to the monitor via a processor. There is a 'digital flexible laryngoscope' available. Clarity of the image is better than that relayed by a fibreoptic bundle; however, failure of any part of the digital system could render the whole scope inoperative, which is not the case with the fibreoptic scope.

HANDLING OF THE INSTRUMENT

The fibreoptic laryngoscope is always best held with the insertion tube straight (Fig. 2.13). This prevents

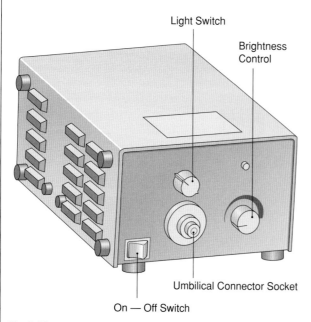

Light Switch

Brightness Control

Umbilical Connector Socket

On — Off Switch

Fig. 2.11
A simple halogen light source. There are usually two lamps, one acting as a spare; hence the 'Light Switch'.

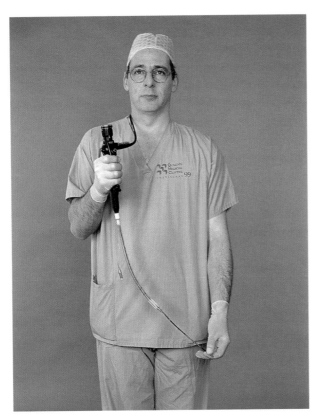

Fig. 2.13
Correct way in which to hold the scope when moving around.
Note the endotracheal tube that has already been loaded onto
the scope and pushed over the stock of the control body.

accidental damage to the insertion tube when moving about and will improve the control over the tip of the instrument during an endoscopy. Excessive bending can stress the fibre bundles and lead to fracture.

It should be appreciated that when the anaesthetist looks down the scope there will be a view over 75–95°. This is the 'field of view', which is dependent upon the type of lens and its seating in the tip of the instrument (Fig. 2.14). It should also be borne in mind that if the lens gets covered in saline or secretions, the angle of view will be diminished until the fluid clears.

DISTAL TIP

Up and down movements

Moving the lever on the control body up and down moves the tip of the scope up and down but remember that it works in reverse, i.e. when the lever is pushed up, the tip will point downwards (Fig. 2.15). The arc that the tip can move through is up to ~260°, depending upon which scope is being used. Scopes also vary as to whether the up and down movements are equal, the up movement frequently being the dominant arc. When buying a scope, try to get one in which the up movement of the tip is the greater, as looking up, or anteriorly, is required more frequently during a fibreoptic laryngoscopy.

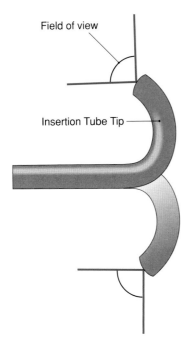

Fig. 2.14
Flexible tip of the fibreoptic laryngoscope.

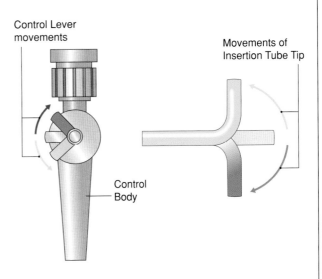

Fig. 2.15
Tip movement as activated by the control lever. Note the reversal of movement.

Side to side movements

Up and to the side

Looking from side to side is a little trickier. There is no mechanism in the fibreoptic laryngoscope that can move the tip of the instrument from side to side (unlike in gastroscopes). If the operator wishes to look right, they must turn the tip of the scope upwards and then twist the control body clockwise (Fig. 2.16). This twist is replicated at the tip and brings the up-bent tip over to the side. At first, as the operator begins to twist clockwise, the view will become up and to the right, and with more twist it will become more and more to the right, and less and less upward, as the tip swings from the vertical to the horizontal. If the index finger of one's left hand is bent to 90°, so that its tip points to the ceiling, and then the wrist is rotated so that the finger is pointing to the right, this action is similar

to the movement of the tip of the laryngoscope. To look left, twist anticlockwise.

The operator can vary how far left or right they view by varying how far the tip is deflected upwards; a 45° up tilt will end up looking left or right at 45° once the insertion tube is twisted through 90° (Fig. 2.17).

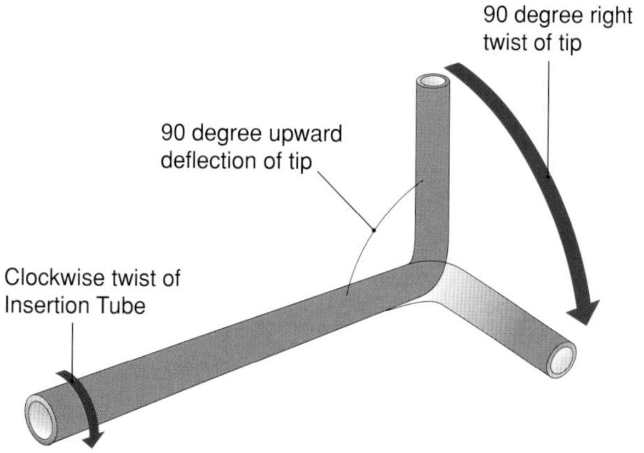

Down and to the side

To look down and to the side, the operator must turn the tip downwards and then twist the control body. Be aware that in the case of downward movement, to look right the control body must be twisted anticlockwise i.e. opposite to the twist that is applied when the tip is upward (Fig. 2.18).

This reversal can make the first few trials with a fibreoptic laryngoscope tricky but after a while the scope movements will become more fluid and will become second nature. Using a finger as a model, as described above, will aid visualisation of the movements of the laryngoscope's tip and show how the reversals work.

Frequently, it will be found that the twist on the control body is not fully reproduced at the tip. This is caused by the scope sticking against something, usually the endotracheal tube wall or the diaphragm of an endoscopy port. To help, the insertion tube can be held with the free hand where it enters the patient or a piece of equipment, and can be gently encouraged to follow the twist of the control body (Fig 2.19). Never be tempted to force the insertion tube if it does not wish to follow the desired twist. This action just risks permanent damage to the fibreoptic bundles, or the essential flexible cover of the insertion tube.

Fig. 2.16
Effect of rotating the insertion tube when the tip is deflected upwards.

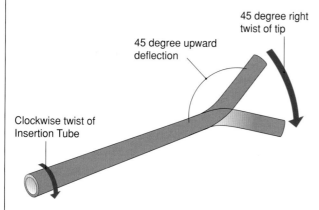

Fig. 2.17
How to look towards the right-hand side.

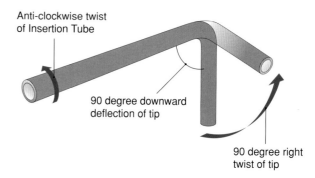

Fig. 2.18
Note how the insertion tube has to be rotated anticlockwise to look right when the tip of the scope is turned downwards.

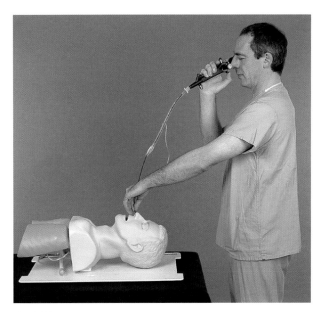

Fig. 2.19
A good position for controlling the tip of the scope.

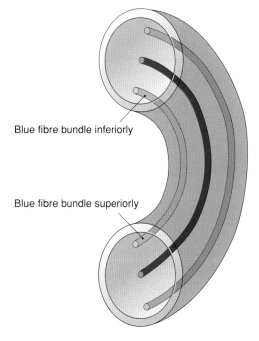

Blue fibre bundle inferiorly

Blue fibre bundle superiorly

Fig. 2.20
Note how the position of the fibre bundles in the viewing bundle reverse their position when approaching the patient from the front. This will invert the image seen at the eyepiece.

FORWARD AND BACKWARD MOVEMENTS

The only other movement is 'forwards and backwards', which is simply accomplished by pushing the scope in and out of the patient or endotracheal tube. Again, gentle encouragement from the free hand often helps, as does good lubrication.

IMAGE INVERSION

The above descriptions hold true if the patient is approached from behind. Unfortunately, things get more complicated when the patient is approached from the front. In this situation, once the tip of the insertion tube has passed into the nasopharynx, the superior part of the endoscopic view will be inferior in the patient (Fig. 2.20) and to look up the lever must be moved up and not down, as previously

described. To look left and right in the patient is no different to that already indicated (when the tip is up, twist clockwise to look to the right in the patient). The best way to appreciate these changes is to try out the movements using a fibreoptic intubation training model, such as the Haridas–Hawkins Trainer, which is described in Chapter 9.

COST

At the time of writing, a new fibreoptic laryngoscope will cost ~£5500–8500 (see glossary). A light source may cost up to £800, while a video camera attachment can be as much as £4000. Over and above this expenditure will be the running costs of the instrument. This aspect will be described in Chapter 8.

3

Indications for fibreoptic intubation

AWAKE INTUBATION

INTUBATION UNDER GENERAL ANAESTHESIA

NASAL INTUBATION

ORAL INTUBATION

CONTRAINDICATIONS TO FIBREOPTIC INTUBATION

ETHICAL CONSIDERATIONS

OTHER USES OF THE FIBREOPTIC LARYNGOSCOPE

Deciding which patients should undergo a fibreoptic intubation is the most crucial part of the technique and common sense is one of the best attributes that a fibreoptic endoscopist can possess. It is fairly easy to decide on a fibreoptic intubation in patients in whom the pathology is gross, as it is easy to decide on a direct laryngoscopy in a normal patient. It is the patient who is considered borderline that presents the greatest difficulty. For this reason many practitioners have tried to dissect the fundamental signs of the difficult intubation so that the anaesthetist may predict which patients will be difficult (see Appendices). Unfortunately, these signs are poor predictors of a difficult intubation when considered in isolation. For example, of all the patients with a Mallampati score (see glossary) of 4, only ~6% will be difficult to intubate, whereas there are patients who score only 1 or 2 and who will be just as difficult. If the results of several of these tests are combined, then prediction of a difficult intubation improves, but it is still far from ideal, with too many false-positives and false-negatives.

There are many conditions known to be associated with difficulty at intubation and these are listed in the Appendices.

AWAKE INTUBATION

Indications

If one is concerned about a potentially difficult airway, it is useful to perform a fibreoptic examination of the airway before finally deciding on the best technique by which to secure it safely. In certain cases it will be decided that an awake tracheostomy is the best choice, while in other cases a normal laryngoscopy under general anaesthesia may be the best option. It should also be borne in mind that if a patient has laryngeal obstruction, the technique chosen should be one with which the anaesthetist is very familiar; these cases are not suitable for the novice.

There are a few simple observations to help the practitioner decide which patients will benefit from an awake procedure (Table 3.1).

If there is uncertainty whether the airway can be maintained after the induction of general anaesthesia, then tracheal intubation should be performed with the patient awake. Some authorities suggest that it is acceptable to perform an inhalational induction of general anaesthesia and to then perform a direct laryngoscopy. If the airway obstructs, it is believed that the patient will awaken, because they can no longer absorb any more anaesthetic gases and that the airway will then open.

Table 3.1. Factors for deciding if a patient is suitable for an awake procedure

If there has been an alteration in the voice
If the patient has stridor
If the patient needs to use their accessory muscles of respiration
If the patient needs to sit up/lean forward to breathe
If the upper airway is deformed
If access to the mouth is denied
If the neck is flexed and fixed
If the patient has signs and symptoms of sleep apnoea
If the patient has had a previous difficult intubation

However, it will be found that when a severely compromised airway obstructs completely, as the airway musculature relaxes, it can fail to re-open, even if no more anaesthetic agent is administered. Surface tension of the upper airway secretions probably plays a part in this failure to regain the airway. Once general anaesthesia has been induced, it is too late to discover that the wrong decision has been made.

If a patient is at a high risk of aspiration of gastric contents, then an awake intubation can be considered. However, it is probably worth leaving the trachea un-anaesthetised so that the patient can still protect their airway to a degree by coughing and turning their head to the side should there be regurgitation of gastric contents.

Awake tracheal intubation can often be achieved in the moribund or comatose patient although the patient may still have some awareness of the procedure.

Some authorities also consider that teaching is an acceptable indication to perform a fibreoptic intubation awake. I cannot agree with this as the patient has no clinical indication to be awake and it is known that some patients will suffer discomfort during the intubation.

The patient with the unstable cervical spine may be intubated awake (see below).

Advantages

The main advantage obtained from using an awake technique to intubate the trachea of a patient with a difficult airway comes from the ability of the patient to maintain their own airway prior to intubation. The tone inherent in the upper airway is preserved and helps to keep the pharynx open. This is the reason why an awake fibreoptic intubation should be chosen in a patient whose airway cannot be guaranteed to be maintained after the loss of consciousness. The patient can also be placed in the position in which they find it easiest to breathe.

Other advantages of this method include having the ability to ask the patient to take a deep breath, which will open the laryngeal inlet and help with the railroading of the endotracheal tube into the trachea. The patient can also swallow troublesome secretions. In addition, with a good local anaesthetic technique, there appears to be little in the way of a hypertensive response to fibreoptic intubation, which is in contrast to a fibreoptic intubation under general anaesthesia. This lack of response is thought to occur because of the neural blockade induced in the upper airway by the local anaesthetic.

Disadvantages

Patients undergoing an awake fibreoptic intubation can experience unpleasant sensations. The application of the local anaesthetic can be unpleasant and make the patient cough, especially if a crico-thyroid stab is performed. The passing of the insertion tube through the upper airway can irritate and railroading the endotracheal tube into the trachea can cause discomfort. All of these sensations are diminished by the use of sedation or opioids and only a small percentage of patients will have any recall of unpleasant feelings if these agents are used. There will always, however, be a small group of patients who will find the technique uncomfortable. This makes good pre-operative counselling, good communication with the patient during the procedure and an excellent local anaesthetic technique essential. Probably the best way to ensure patient compliance is to explain just why an awake technique is necessary. When the patient understands that the technique has been chosen with their survival as the prime consideration, then most people tolerate an awake fibreoptic intubation very well.

Young children and uncooperative patients are not suitable for an awake fibreoptic intubation.

INTUBATION UNDER GENERAL ANAESTHESIA

Indications

Most practitioners will opt for a general anaesthetic technique in patients in whom it is reasonably certain that ventilation of the lungs can be maintained after the loss of consciousness. This avoids discomfort for the patient and anxiety in the anaesthetist. No one likes to see a patient suffer, least of all unnecessarily. However, do not feel that a general anaesthetic must be performed in a patient with a difficult airway because of the unpleasantness of the procedure when awake. These feelings pale into insignificance when compared with the consequences of the total loss of the airway when general anaesthesia is induced.

The patient with an unstable cervical spine is a difficult airway management problem and needs very careful assessment before deciding on the best technique for intubating the trachea. The main problem concerns movement of the neck during the procedure caused by the technique itself, and spontaneous movement in the form of bucking and coughing. At present, there is no definitive way in which to secure the airway of this type of patient and fibreoptic intubation is only one of the methods advocated. The main considerations involve the speed at which intubation is required and whether to perform the procedure awake or anaesthetised. In the emergency situation, when intubation is required very quickly, fibreoptic intubation is not the technique of choice; oral or nasal intubation under general anaesthesia with in-line stabilisation of the neck, or a surgical airway, are more appropriate.

In a patient with an unstable cervical fracture, it is wise to perform the fibreoptic intubation under general anaesthesia, unless there are other compounding factors involving the airway. This is especially true for the patient who already has evidence of spinal cord compression, because any movement in such a patient can have disastrous consequences. A slow inhalational induction can be performed via a nasal airway (after applying local anaesthetic to the nose) using a volatile agent such as sevoflurane in oxygen. A small dose of fentanyl helps prevent upper airway irritation and coughing during this part of the procedure. Just prior to passing the vocal cords with the insertion tube (and when one is confident that this and railroading of the endotracheal tube into the trachea will be straightforward), the patient's muscles can be fully paralysed with a non-depolarising muscle relaxant such as rocuronium, and alfentanil can be given to obtain potent suppression of the airway reflexes. This will prevent any coughing or movement as the insertion tube is passed into the trachea and the endotracheal tube is railroaded. The problem with this technique is the diminution in the size of the airway with induction of anaesthesia, which then has the potential to obstruct. It must be remembered that head and neck manoeuvres and jaw thrust can cause cervical spine movement and that laryngeal and cricoid cartilage manipulations may be just as dangerous. Anterior tongue traction may cause less neck movement if performed carefully and will

help to re-open the airway. If this fails, the patient can still be intubated by direct laryngoscopy with in-line stabilisation of the neck.

Some authorities use awake fibreoptic intubation in patients with a cervical fracture in the belief that even if the patient coughs or gags, muscle tone will prevent any movement of the spine and damage to the spinal cord, and that the airway will be protected if regurgitation of gastric contents occurs. However, it is known that severe coughing can result from both the 'spray as you go' and crico-thyroid stab local anaesthetic techniques, and that laryngeal spasm has been reported in the awake patient undergoing fibreoptic intubation.

General anaesthesia is also indicated for a patient with a normal airway when a fibreoptic teaching session has been planned. However, ensure that the patient has given informed consent for the teaching element of the proposed technique. Most children will also require a general anaesthetic.

The only other positive indication for a general anaesthetic technique is when the patient refuses to undergo awake intubation. The practitioner should explain to the patient that there will be increased risk to their wellbeing if a general anaesthetic is administered.

Advantages

The main advantage to general anaesthesia is the removal of awareness for the patient and the removal of any risk of movement in spinal cases. It also allows the anaesthetist to practice the technique of fibreoptic intubation on patients with normal airways. In this situation the airway can be manipulated by dropping the jaw and manipulating the neck a little, which will make the airway more difficult to negotiate. Total intravenous anaesthesia is ideal in this situation.

Disadvantages

The main disadvantage of general anaesthesia is the narrowing of the airway that occurs with this technique, which is due to a diminution in the tone of the airway musculature as anaesthesia is induced (Figs. 3.1 and 3.2). This can make fibreoptic intubation more difficult and there is always the risk that the airway will be lost completely as it narrows. Another disadvantage is the increased salivation that occurs with general anaesthesia, although an intravenous antisialagogue (see glossary) given a few minutes before helps. Applying suction to the pharyngeal secretions prior to endoscopy is also beneficial.

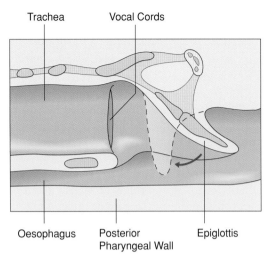

Fig. 3.1
Representation of the larynx showing how the epiglottis tends towards the posterior pharyngeal wall following induction of general anaesthesia.

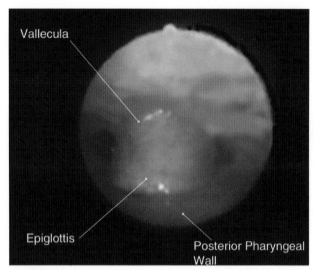

Fig. 3.2
Endoscopic view of a floppy or 'curtain' epiglottis abutting the posterior pharyngeal wall. This image was taken with some jaw thrust already applied.

NASAL INTUBATION

Indications

There are three reasons why fibreoptic intubation via the nasal route may be chosen. First, the operation may require a nasal tube, e.g. dental or maxillofacial procedures. Second, one may wish to perform a nasal intubation because it is usually easier and has a higher success rate compared with an oral approach. Finally, there may be poor access to the oral cavity, as in temporomandibular ankylosis.

Advantages

The main advantage of a nasal approach for fibreoptic intubation is the route which the scope must take to reach the laryngeal inlet. It will frequently be found that once the insertion tube has passed into the pharynx, the laryngeal inlet or epiglottis will be directly in front (Fig. 3.3).

This straight approach to the larynx and trachea brings the added advantage that the endotracheal tube passes more easily into the trachea during railroading (Fig. 3.4). The insertion tube also tends to stay midline when using this approach, which

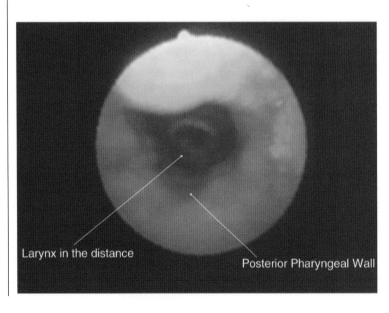

Fig. 3.3
Typical endoscopic view of the larynx from the nasopharynx.

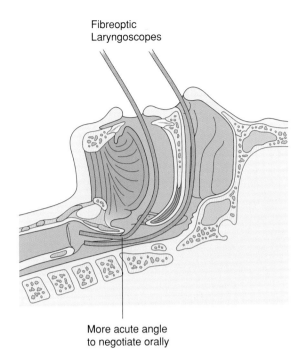

Fibreoptic
Laryngoscopes

More acute angle
to negotiate orally

Fig. 3.4
The better route taken by the insertion tube in a nasal
approach.

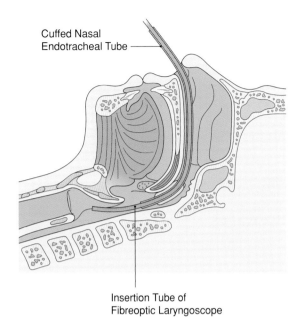

Cuffed Nasal
Endotracheal Tube

Insertion Tube of
Fibreoptic Laryngoscope

Fig. 3.5
How the endotracheal tube can act as a clean conduit for the
insertion tube.

makes the endoscopy even easier. Another benefit of the nasal approach is the stability of the endotracheal tube once it has been secured in position, because the tube is supported by the walls of the nasal cavities.

Disadvantages

The main problem with nasal intubation is bleeding. It is estimated that between 8 and 22% of nasal fibreoptic intubations cause an epistaxis; however, the passage of the insertion tube itself should rarely cause this problem. If there is significant bleeding, it can make the intubation difficult as it can obscure the view and can also make the patient cough and feel nauseated if it is an awake procedure. This can make all efforts to intubate the trachea a fruitless exercise. The use of vasoconstrictors, choosing the most patent nostril and the use of a warm or flexible endotracheal tube all help minimise this problem. Usually, bleeding is caused by the passage of the endotracheal tube through the nostril. Some practitioners suggest sizing the nostril with nasopharyngeal airways first, but this can cause bleeding itself. A better solution is to pass the endotracheal tube through the more patent nostril and into the pharynx and to then pass the scope through the endotracheal tube. The tube not only

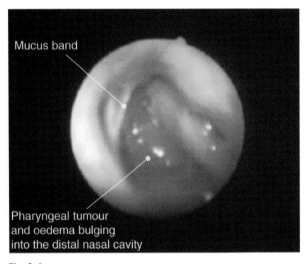

Mucus band

Pharyngeal tumour
and oedema bulging
into the distal nasal cavity

Fig. 3.6
Endoscopic image of part of a large tumour/oedematous mass
completely occluding both distal nasal cavities.

helps tamponade any bleeding points, but also protects the scope from any blood (Fig. 3.5).

Occasionally the nasal cavities may be so restricted or blocked by a tumour or oedema that passing a nasal tube may be impossible (Fig. 3.6). Therefore, it is wise to inspect both nasal cavities with the fibreoptic laryngoscope before performing the full endoscopy. It is frustrating, embarrassing and potentially dangerous to find that the endotracheal tube cannot be passed through the nose after the scope is in the trachea.

Passage of the endotracheal tube through the nose can cause discomfort in the awake patient and there is a small incidence of nasal soreness post-operatively.

ORAL INTUBATION

Advantages

The main advantages in using an oral approach for intubation are, that there is less chance of causing bleeding and no nasal soreness post-operatively. It is also used when the nasal route is not an option.

Disadvantages

An oral fibreoptic intubation succeeds less frequently than the nasal route because of the angle between the oral cavity and the laryngeal inlet and trachea. This angle is a lot greater than that negotiated in a nasal approach. This problem is made worse if there is little space between the posterior pharyngeal wall and the epiglottis, if the tongue is large or if the head cannot be extended, which helps straighten out the angle. In addition if the angle is too great it may be impossible to reach the larynx, which can be sitting above the tip of the fibreoptic laryngoscope but cannot be reached. It is also more difficult to keep the insertion tube in the midline using the oral route.

Several oral fibreoptic-intubating aids have been designed to overcome these problems (Fig. 3.7).

They are made so that the insertion tube will have already negotiated the sharp angle in the upper airway by the time the scope has reached the end of the oral airway; the larynx should then be directly in front of the tip of the scope. These aids also help to keep the base of the tongue away from the scope. Some will allow the passage of an endotracheal tube through them, while others are removed from around the insertion tube before railroading. Despite this, the endotracheal tube is known to 'hang up' more frequently during railroading when the oral route is used.

An awake procedure via the oral route may also be more difficult for the patient, due to stimulation of the gag reflex. There is also the added risk to the fibreoptic laryngoscope from biting.

CONTRAINDICATIONS TO FIBREOPTIC INTUBATION

The few contraindications to performing a fibreoptic intubation are:

- Patient refusal
- Need to secure the airway immediately
- Lack of the other skills necessary to manage a difficult airway
- Lack of training in the technique of fibreoptic intubation

Relative contraindications include:

- Profuse bleeding in the airway
- Partial laryngeal obstruction (tumour or epiglottitis)
- Massive facial injury
- Basilar skull fracture (nasal route)

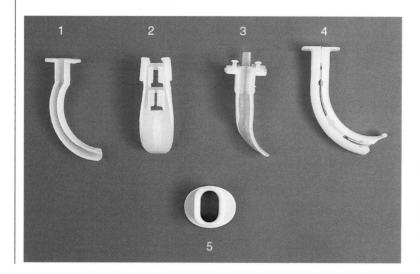

Fig. 3.7
Five oral airways: 1, Guedel cut in half; 2, Ovassapian; 3, VBM; 4, Berman; and 5, oral bite block that can protect the fibreoptic laryngoscope during an awake oral intubation if no other airway is available. The oral bite block will allow a 9-mm endotracheal tube and its connector to pass through.

ETHICAL CONSIDERATIONS

Ethically, one should ensure that that the patient is not harmed and that they will benefit from a proposed procedure. Therefore, any potentially harmful or unpleasant procedure, from which the patient will derive no benefit, is unethical. Fibreoptic intubation in a normal patient under general anaesthesia is justified because there is no evidence to suggest that it is any more dangerous than a normal intubation. In fact, it has been shown to be less traumatic than direct laryngoscopy. Therefore, using this technique on the normal patient to teach the technique and to maintain a practitioner's skills is ethical. One could argue that as a fibreoptic endoscopist, one is morally obliged to use the technique. However, when there is no medical indication for an intubation to be performed awake, an awake fibreoptic intubation is hard to justify.

OTHER USES OF THE FIBREOPTIC LARYNGOSCOPE

The fibreoptic laryngoscope can be used for purposes other than tracheal intubation:

- Checking the position of an endotracheal tube
- Checking the patency of an endotracheal tube
- Placement of double lumen tubes and endobronchial blockers
- Examination of the upper airway
- Examination of the nares before nasal intubation
- Placement of difficult nasogastric tubes

4

Local anaesthesia of the upper airway

INNERVATION OF THE UPPER AIRWAY

STRUCTURES REQUIRING ANAESTHESIA FOR AWAKE INTUBATION

AGENTS USED FOR AIRWAY ANAESTHESIA

TECHNIQUES

INNERVATION OF THE UPPER AIRWAY

Sensation to the oral and nasal cavities, the roof of the nasopharynx and part of the soft palate is provided by the trigeminal nerve. The glossopharyngeal nerve supplies the posterior third of the tongue, the posterior soft palate, the superior aspect of the epiglottis and remaining nasopharynx and oropharynx. Further down the airway the vagus nerve supplies the larynx via the internal laryngeal branch of the superior laryngeal nerve. This supplies the laryngopharynx, piriform fossae and the larynx above the false cords. The rest of the larynx (the false cords and below) is supplied by the recurrent laryngeal nerve, which also supplies the upper trachea.

STRUCTURES REQUIRING ANAESTHESIA FOR AWAKE INTUBATION

If the nasal route is used, then the nasal cavity and nasopharynx must be anaesthetised and a vasoconstricter applied to the mucosa to minimise the risk of bleeding. If the oral route is used, then the middle and posterior thirds of the tongue must be anaesthetised.

The soft palate, posterior oropharynx, epiglottis, larynx and trachea must be anaesthetised in either situation (Fig. 4.1).

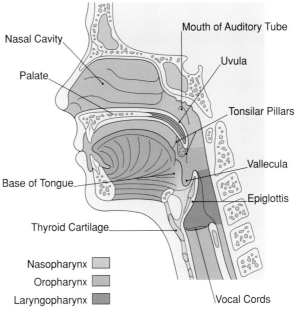

Fig. 4.1
Anatomy of the airway as far as the larynx.

AGENTS USED FOR AIRWAY ANAESTHESIA

The anaesthetic agents most commonly used are:

- Lidocaine
- Cocaine

True allergy to local anaesthetics is rare but would preclude topical anaesthesia of the airway.

Lidocaine

Lidocaine is by far the most commonly used agent in the UK. It is rapidly acting and produces anaesthesia in ~1 minute following its topical application to mucous membranes. Its effects last for ~30 minute. It is available in concentrations of 2–10% and can be used for both nerve blocks and topical anaesthesia. The maximum recommended dose is 3 mg/kg (see glossary); however, as much as 11 mg/kg has been used and, in almost all reported cases, the peak plasma concentrations have been below that recommended for the therapeutic control of ventricular arrhythmias. This is probably due to the loss of the majority of the drug in the saliva, which is swallowed, with subsequent deactivation of the drug by hepatic metabolism.

Cocaine

Cocaine is available as a 4–10% paste and is used for nasal anaesthesia because it has both local anaesthetic and vasoconstrictor properties. The anaesthetic effect is very rapid in onset, while its vasoconstrictor action takes between 5 and 10 minutes to appear.

Cocaine selectively inhibits the re-uptake of norepinephrine, which makes it pro-arrhythmic. It has been implicated in the causation of myocardial infarction following topical application and should therefore be used with caution. The maximum recommended dose is 1.5 mg/kg when applied to the nasal mucosa.

Cocaine should not be used if the patient has porphyria.

TECHNIQUES

Before applying any of the techniques described below, the monitors should be attached to the patient and an intravenous cannula must be inserted. The operator should also have knowledge of the signs of local anaesthetic toxicity and its treatment.

Techniques to anaesthetise the airway include:

- Topical application
- Crico-thyroid stab
- Internal laryngeal nerve block
- Glossopharyngeal nerve block

Topical anaesthesia

Topical anaesthesia is the commonest method used to anaesthetise the pharynx, larynx and trachea, and is the only way to anaesthetise the nose. The quality of anaesthesia is improved if an antisialagogue is given before the application of the local anaesthetic. Glycopyrronium bromide is better than atropine in this regard and it begins to have an effect in 2–15 minutes depending upon the patient. It should be noted that enhanced absorption of the local anaesthetic occurs if a drying agent is used.

Nose

Before the application of the local anaesthetic to the nasal mucosa, it is best to apply a vasoconstrictor. Xylometazoline and oxymetazoline are very useful and available as sprays, but ephedrine can be diluted to 5 mg/ml and applied with a 'swab on a stick'. Remember that all three drugs are sympathomimetics and should, therefore, never be used in patients receiving mono-amine oxidase inhibitors, or if cocaine is to be used.

The local anaesthetic solution can be sprayed into each nostril or applied as a gel/paste to the nasal mucosa using a microbiological 'swab on a stick' (Fig 5.1), the gel or paste being applied gently in a circular motion and being worked deeper and deeper into the nostril. If time is taken over this stage of the procedure, the patient will feel minimal discomfort. Once the nostril is anaesthetised, a lidocaine spray can be used deep in the nostril, which will help to anaesthetise the pharynx. The patient should be warned that the taste of the spray can be unpleasant. It is advisable to avoid using the 10% lidocaine spray in the nose as it can cause pain.

Pharynx

Lidocaine can be sprayed into the pharynx via the mouth or via the nostril, as described above, using either a commercially available 10% spray or an atomiser with 2–4% lidocaine solution. A nebuliser with 4 ml 2–4% lidocaine can also be used either as the primary technique or as a supplementary method of anaesthesia, as can gargling with 20–30 ml (see glossary) of a 2% solution two or three times; get the patient to spit out any excess solution to avoid overdosage of lidocaine.

Many practitioners rely on the 'spray as you go' technique once the nose or the mouth is anaesthetised. With this technique a local anaesthetic solution is injected down the working channel of the fibreoptic laryngoscope under direct vision (Fig. 4.2); 3–4 ml is used on each occasion, sometimes

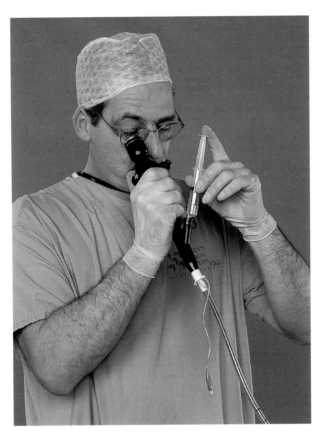

Fig. 4.2
Note how the operator continues to observe as the local anaesthetic solution is injected. This is to ensure its correct placement.

with the addition of an equal volume of air to help force the solution down the channel and to help atomise it as it leaves the tip of the scope. The patient often coughs as the spray hits un-anaesthetised areas of the airway, but this reaction soon subsides. Once an area is anaesthetised, the scope can be moved further into the airway to spray the next region. It is a good idea to spray into the pharynx just as it is entered as some of it will reach the larynx directly or be carried there by the patient's inspirations.

Whichever method is used, it is wise to wait for a short period for the anaesthetic to work before proceeding.

Larynx and trachea

These structures can both be anaesthetised topically by the 'spray as you go' technique or by a crico-thyroid injection of local anaesthetic.

'Spray as you go'
The tip of the insertion tube must be close to the larynx to ensure the correct placement of the local

anaesthetic solution. Once the scope has passed through the vocal cords, the upper trachea can be sprayed. Coughing helps to distribute the solution further down the trachea.

Crico-thyroid injection
In this very useful technique, local anaesthetic is deposited in the tracheal lumen by an injection through the crico-thyroid membrane. Coughing then distributes the anaesthetic up and down the trachea and onto the larynx.

A 10-ml syringe fitted with a 22-gauge needle is filled with 4 ml of 2% plain lidocaine. The needle is then passed through the crico-thyroid membrane perpendicularly. Aspiration of air confirms entry into the trachea and advancement of the needle is halted at this point to prevent breaching the posterior tracheal wall and oesophagus (Figs. 4.3 and 4.4). The needle shaft is then held firmly at the point where it enters the skin and the patient is asked to breathe out and hold their breath. The contents of the syringe is then injected rapidly into the trachea. The instant that the injection ceases, the needle and syringe must be withdrawn rapidly. As a reflex, the patient will inspire deeply and then cough, which distributes the local anaesthetic up and down the trachea and onto the larynx.

Bleeding, infection and mediastinitis have all been reported as complications of this technique. Because a significant number of patients will cough severely during this technique, its use is inadvisable in the patient with the unstable cervical spine.

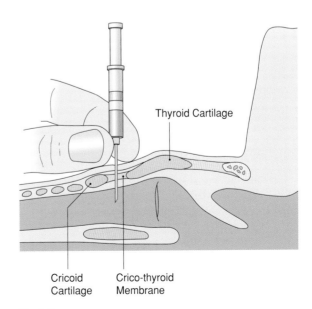

Thyroid Cartilage

Cricoid Cartilage   Crico-thyroid Membrane

Fig. 4.3
Completed insertion of the needle through the crico-thyroid membrane. Note the firm grip on the needle where it enters the skin.

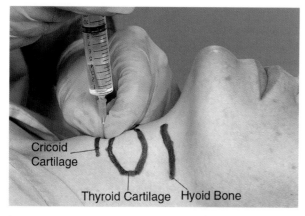

Fig. 4.4
Crico-thyroid stab: note how the head is extended and how the operator has gripped the needle firmly at the level of the skin to prevent it from passing deeper into the trachea when the patient coughs.

Contraindications to this technique include:

- Infection at the site of injection
- Coagulopathy
- Inability to locate the crico-thyroid membrane (obesity /deformity)
- Tumour/stenosis at or close to injection site
- Patient refusal

Nerve blocks

Nerve blocks can be used as the sole technique to anaesthetise the pharynx or laryngopharynx, or as supplements to topical anaesthesia. However, their use is optional and usually unnecessary. They need to be performed bilaterally.

It is possible to block the following nerves:

- Internal laryngeal nerve
- Glossopharyngeal nerve

Internal laryngeal nerve blocks

The internal laryngeal nerve block has in the past been referred to as the superior laryngeal nerve block. However, it is the internal branch of the superior laryngeal nerve that is anaesthetised in the techniques described below.

Blocking the internal laryngeal nerves will provide anaesthesia to the following structures:

- Laryngeal mucosa down to the vocal cords
- Laryngeal surface of the epiglottis
- Piriform fossae

The internal laryngeal nerve runs close to the hyoid

bone and under the piriform fossae and can be blocked in either position.

Bradycardia and severe hypotension have been reported following this block, so it is advisable to use it on selected cases only.

Hyoid position

This block can be performed in the sitting or supine position, but in either case it is good to have the head extended and it is also wise to ask that the patient neither talks nor swallows while the block is being performed. The hyoid bone should be stabilised by gently pressing it from the opposite side so that it becomes more prominent on the injection side. The surface landmark for this block is the greater cornu of the hyoid bone (Fig. 4.5).

A 22–25-gauge 3-cm needle with a 5-ml syringe attached, is advanced perpendicularly to the skin to hit the hyoid at the position of the greater cornu, or 1 cm anterior to it (Fig. 4.6). Having hit the bone, the needle is carefully 'walked' off the inferior edge of the bone and passed just through the thyro-hyoid membrane; a 'give' may be felt as the needle passes through the membrane — stop at 2 cm if this is not felt. Local anaesthetic (1–3 ml, use a high concentration if possible) is deposited in this position after aspirating to make sure that the pharynx has not been entered.

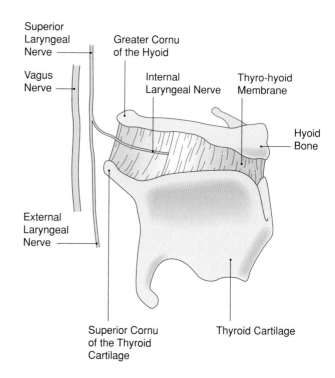

Fig. 4.5
Course of the 'laryngeal' nerves.

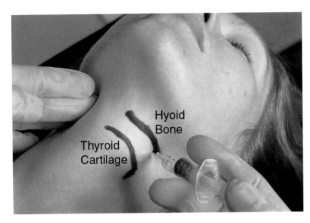

Fig. 4.6
Internal laryngeal nerve block: note how the operator's free
hand displaces the hyoid towards the block side to make it
more prominent.

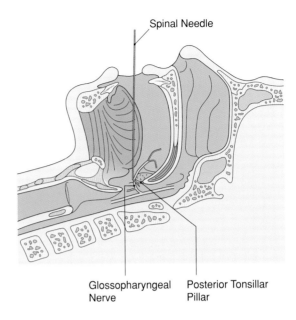

Fig. 4.7
Injection position for a glossopharyngeal nerve block.

The block can also be performed by identifying
the superior cornu of the thyroid cartilage (or 1 cm
anterior to it) and walking superiorly off it, but
avoid injection through the thyroid cartilage, which
could cause swelling around the vocal cords.

If the nerve is hit, pain is referred to the ear. In
addition, if the local anaesthetic diffuses back to
involve the superior laryngeal nerve or its external
branch, then the patient may experience temporary
hoarseness of the voice. This is due to paralysis of
the crico-thyroid muscle, which normally tenses the
vocal cords. In the severely compromised airway,
functioning of this muscle may be important.

Piriform fossa position
The internal laryngeal nerve runs just under the
mucous membrane covering the piriform fossa,
where it is easily blocked by applying a cotton wool
ball soaked in 2% lidocaine by means of a pair of
Krause's forceps. These are passed through the
mouth after anterior tongue traction has been
applied. Keeping to the lateral pharyngeal wall
follow it down into the piriform fossa. A fullness
should be felt if the thyro-hyoid membrane is
palpated from the outside in a lateral position. The
local anaesthetic needs to be applied for 1–2
minutes, and sometimes longer.

The oropharynx and the posterior two-thirds
of the tongue need to be anaesthetised before
performing this block, or the patient will feel
discomfort and may retch.

Glossopharyngeal nerve block

If 2–3 ml of local anaesthetic solution are
placed behind the posterior tonsillar pillar at its
midpoint or at its base, at a depth of 1 cm, the
glossopharyngeal nerve will be blocked. If
performed bilaterally the following regions will be
anaesthetised:

- Posterior third of the tongue
- Pharyngeal surface of the epiglottis
- Tonsillar region
- Oropharynx

The tongue and tonsillar pillars need to be
anaesthetised before performing the block, which
can be done topically.

A 7–8-cm needle is required with the last 1 cm
bent at ~45° (a 22-gauge spinal needle is good
for this Fig. 4.7). Depress the tongue with a normal
laryngoscope and perform the block after aspirating
for blood. Be careful not to go too deep as the
carotid artery is nearby.

Unfortunately use of this technique results in
muscular paralysis of the base of the tongue and the
pharynx, which can precipitate loss of the airway.
The gag reflex is also abolished and the block is best
used only if this reflex is causing a problem with the
endoscopy.

5

Conduct of fibreoptic intubation

Whichever method of anaesthesia is adopted for intubation, careful pre-operative assessment accomplishes several useful functions:

- Elucidation of the nature and severity of airway problems
- Assessment of the patient's medical, physiological and psychological status
- Reassurance of the patient
- Opportunity to prescribe appropriate premedication

The nature of the airway problem and the anaesthetist's experience and training will, to some extent, guide the method chosen for intubation. Severe anatomical abnormalities, inflammation around the airway or an uncooperative patient render the performance of local anaesthetic nerve blocks more difficult and will therefore favour a 'spray as you go' technique. It may be found that when the patient is asked to breathe through each nostril in turn, both nostrils are occluded, which will dictate that an oral approach is necessary.

The presence of severe associated heart disease or anxiety favours the use of a sedative premedicant, but not if the airway is so compromised that premedication would be dangerous. An antisialagogue can help prevent any problems with secretions obscuring the endoscopic view. However, patients do not like drying agents and their use in conjunction with a local anaesthetic lozenge must be timed carefully as it is impossible to dissolve anything in a dry mouth. Finally, premedication should not be a substitute for a clear, reasoned explanation delivered in a patient and sympathetic manner.

It is the author's practice to omit all premedication wherever possible and to give intravenous glycopyrronium bromide (antisialagogue) as soon as the patient arrives in the anaesthetic room. This can be followed by the careful titration of sedatives as appropriate and under careful observation. This negates the twin effects of variable gastrointestinal absorption and inter-patient variation in response to sedation. The combination of fentanyl and midazolam is well proven in this regard and inadvertent overdosage can be reversed with the opiate antagonist naloxone, and the benzodiazepine antagonist, flumazanil.

If cocaine is used for nasal anaesthesia, then other vasoconstrictors are not necessary and may be dangerous.

PATIENT PREPARATION

From the foregoing it can be deduced that the patient should be relaxed and calm before either local or general anaesthesia. An electrocardiogram, a non-invasive blood pressure machine and a pulse oximeter should be connected to the patient, even if intubation is to be performed awake. A capnograph should be available to help confirm the placement of the endotracheal tube within the trachea.

The anaesthetist and assistant (who should ideally be conversant with fibreoptic intubation) should be as appropriately prepared as the patient. All the equipment required must be present and in working order. Thorough checks before commencement of anaesthesia enhance safety and also save any potential embarrassment. For equipment necessary for a safe fibreoptic intubation, see Chapter 8.

AWAKE INTUBATION

What follows is a description of the author's preferred method for intubating the awake patient. It is not necessarily the best method for every anaesthetist; that is only arrived at through trial and practice.

The patient arrives unpremedicated in the anaesthetic room. An intravenous cannula is inserted into a suitable vein and 5 μg/kg body weight glycopyrronium bromide is administered intravenously and a vasoconstrictor applied to the nostrils (if cocaine is not going to be used).

At this stage there should be a second anaesthetist to provide any sedation and to observe and interpret changes in the patient's vital signs. It cannot be over-emphasised that it is impossible to fully monitor a patient while looking down an optical instrument. At this stage the administration of local anaesthetic may commence.

Nasal route

Lidocaine gel or 4% cocaine paste is slowly applied to the nose in a circular motion, working backward with a 'swab on a stick' until it impinges on the posterior wall of the nasopharynx. Microbiological swabs are good for this because they are several centimetres long and can reach the nasopharynx (Fig. 5.1). There is little to be gained from rushing, as the effect of the local anaesthetic will increase over the next few minutes and one of the most important factors in obtaining a successful awake fibreoptic intubation is the quality of the anaesthesia.

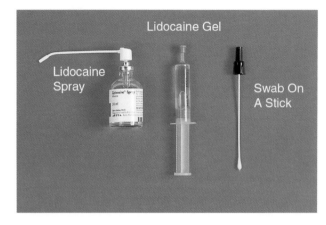

Fig. 5.1
Equipment required to anaesthetise the nose and nasopharynx.

Next, spray local anaesthetic deep into the back of the nose and ask the patient to swallow any that reaches the oropharynx. It is advisable to warn the patient that they may get a nasty taste in the back of the mouth.

The patient should then be asked to sit up and open their mouth as wide as is comfortable so that the back of the throat can be sprayed with lidocaine. Lidocaine 2% is adequate, but commercially available sprays can deliver a 10% solution, so care must be taken not to overdose the patient with this type of high-concentration spray.

The final procedure that completes local anaesthesia is a crico-thyroid stab, which will anaesthetise the trachea, inferior larynx and possibly parts of the pharynx through droplet spread (see Chapter 4).

At this stage there is a dry-mouthed patient in whom the upper airway as far as the lower trachea should be numb. The entire process, if handled slowly and gently, will have been accomplished without much discomfort. However, the insertion of the fibreoptic laryngoscope or endotracheal tube into the upper airway can be uncomfortable, particularly when the endotracheal tube passes through the nose and larynx, and especially in an anxious patient or in the hands of an inexperienced practitioner. Judicious doses of fentanyl (50–200 μg, see glossary) and droperidol (1–2 mg), given incrementally, can make the whole event more comfortable. Midazolam is a short-acting benzodiazepine that can be used instead of droperidol and has the added advantage that it is reversible.

Position the patient so that the head and neck are in the neutral position, and stand behind the patient. Insert an endotracheal tube (lubricated with lidocaine gel) through the nose as far as the

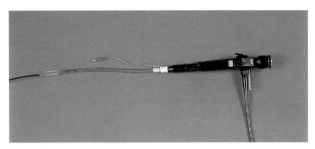

Fig. 5.2
Fibreoptic laryngoscope with an endotracheal tube loaded onto
the stock of the control body before endoscopy.

oropharynx. If the endotracheal tube is not passed
through the nose before endoscopy, ensure that it is
loaded onto the fibreoptic laryngoscope before
starting (Fig. 5.2).

The fibreoptic laryngoscope is now advanced
through the endotracheal tube (or nostril) while
observing the endoscopic view. As the tip of the
scope exits from the endotracheal tube the glottis or
epiglottis will come into view, provided that there
has been no deviation from the midline. The scope
is moved gently forward keeping away from any
mucosal surfaces, blood or secretions. Frequently the
tip does not need to be manipulated very much,
until it needs to be directed beneath the epiglottis
and through the laryngeal inlet. When the larynx sits
~2 cm away from the tip of the scope, a syringe
containing 4 ml 2% lidocaine and 6 ml air should
be rapidly evacuated into the injection port of the
fibreoptic laryngoscope. The air forces the local
anaesthetic out of the working channel and helps to
atomise it. Ideally, this should be done with the
vocal cords in view and the patient should be
warned that the injection will provoke a cough. If
the local anaesthetic is not seen to spray the cords
and no coughing is heard, then it is usually best to
repeat the injection before advancing the tip of the
scope through the larynx and giving a further 4 ml
into the trachea. Again, the patient will cough and
should be warned of this.

If it is difficult to get the tip of the scope to pass
under the epiglottis or through the larynx, ask the
patient to take a deep breath or to put out their
tongue, which can open up the airway and give a
better view.

Once through the vocal cords, the tip of the
insertion tube should be advanced as far as the mid-
trachea, confirming in the process that the tracheal
rings and carina can be seen. The endotracheal tube
can then be railroaded gently over the insertion tube
and down through the pharynx, laryngeal inlet and
into the trachea, with the insertion tube acting as a
lubricated stylet or bougie. It is often best to do this

during a deep breath, which widens the vocal cords,
and while gently rotating the endotracheal tube so
that the tip of the tube does not impinge or 'hang
up' (see glossary) on any part of the larynx. Gentle
pressure on the thyroid cartilage sometimes helps.
The position of the tip of the endotracheal tube (at
the mid-tracheal position) can be verified before
withdrawing the scope. Further verification of the
position of the tube should be obtained using a
capnograph or by feeling the airflow though the
endotracheal tube. It is now safe to induce general
anaesthesia.

Oral route

Anaesthetising the tongue and oropharynx is
achieved in a variety of ways. The easiest is simply
to spray the tongue with 2% lidocaine using either
a simple atomiser, spray or nebuliser. Asking the
patient to gargle with 2% aqueous lidocaine gel
helps complete the task. A crico-thyroid stab and a
top-up to the anaesthesia by spraying the larynx and
trachea are still required. Confirmation of adequate
anaesthesia is offered by the patient's acceptance of
an oral airway without discomfort.

Once good anaesthesia has been established, a
'fibreoptic intubating airway' should be inserted in
the same manner as a Guedel airway. These airways
are split or open along one surface, so that the
airway can be removed from around the insertion
tube before railroading the endotracheal tube. With
some airways it is possible to railroad an
endotracheal tube through them and it is best to
smear these airways with lidocaine gel before use. If
one of these intubating airways is not available,
cutting a wide slit in the lateral or posterior surface
can modify a Guedel type airway. Be careful not to
leave sharp edges as these can damage the scope's
covering.

Once the airway is comfortably in place, the
technique is similar to the nasal approach. With oral
intubation, a suitable endotracheal tube needs to be
placed over the lubricated insertion tube and pushed
gently over or taped onto the stock of the control
body of the scope. The insertion tube is then
inserted gently through the intubating airway. It is
essential to remain in the midline and the split
airway helps with this. It will be found that as the
scope leaves the airway its tip may need to be flexed
to bring the epiglottis into view, and sometimes it
will be found that the tip of the intubating airway
has gone above the epiglottis and into the vallecula.
If so, it needs to be withdrawn until it is clear of the
epiglottis. A deep breath at this stage can help
visualise things better.

The tip of the insertion tube is passed through the larynx and the scope advanced up to the mid-tracheal position as before, remembering to spray the appropriate structures with local anaesthetic. Once the tip of the scope is at the mid-tracheal position, the split oral airway can be removed and the endotracheal tube gently railroaded down through the larynx and into the trachea. Again the patient can be asked to take a deep breath to facilitate this. Confirmation of the position of the tube is as described above.

If at any time visualisation of the anatomy is lost, the scope should be withdrawn slowly to a midline position until the anatomy becomes clearer. It is also useful to remember that the sharp angle that needs to be negotiated in an oral intubation can be lessened by extending the head and neck by removing the pillow or by placing the pillow under the shoulders.

INTUBATION UNDER GENERAL ANAESTHESIA

The preparation and equipment required for fibreoptic intubation under general anaesthesia are the same as for local anaesthesia. This includes attaching the monitors to the patient and the placement of a cannula into a vein prior to commencing anaesthesia.

Techniques have been devised for administering a general anaesthetic safely for fibreoptic intubation. In the end the technique of choice is often a matter of personal preference, experience, and the patient's physiognomy and pathology. Oral or nasal intubation is possible and the patient may be allowed to breathe spontaneously or the muscles may be paralysed and the lungs artificially ventilated. A drying agent is especially useful if irritant volatile agents are to be used.

Many practitioners faced with a difficult airway use a gaseous induction. The patient can be left breathing spontaneously or the airway can be gently tested to see if intermittent positive pressure ventilation with a mask is possible. If it is, then a total intravenous technique can be used while intubation is accomplished. It is possible to maintain anaesthesia using a nasal airway connected directly to an anaesthetic circuit while intubation takes place down the other nostril. Alternatively, a specially modified mask known as an endoscopy mask can be used. It has a hole in a membrane to allow the passage of the scope and the following endotracheal tube. Great caution and experience is required if muscle relaxants are to be used before intubation and a suitable period of pre-oxygenation with 100%

oxygen is mandatory.

More recently, the use of a laryngeal mask airway (LMA) as an aid to fibreoptic intubation has been described and may be especially useful for the inexperienced practitioner to help minimise any period of apnoea (see Chapter 9). Unfortunately, some of these techniques require the LMA cuff to be cut and resealed with silicone glue.

Passage of the scope through the airway is not dissimilar to the awake method. However, it may be necessary for an assistant to perform various manoeuvres to open the airway. This is especially true if the epiglottis approximates the posterior pharyngeal wall because of the loss of tone in the airway musculature that occurs on induction of anaesthesia. These manoeuvres may include jaw thrust (Fig. 5.3), anterior tongue traction, laryngeal lift or even the insertion of a normal laryngoscope to displace the epiglottis anteriorly (see Chapter 7). Under these circumstances, nasal intubation is often easier because in the anaesthetised patient the tongue tends to fall backwards, obscuring the view of the larynx when approached orally. However, if the oral route is chosen, an oral intubating airway is especially useful when a general anaesthetic technique is used.

Experienced practitioners rarely use general anaesthesia for patients with a very difficult airway because haemaglobin oxygen desaturation commonly occurs and the procedure is usually more difficult — and dangerous in extreme cases. However, a patient in whom tracheal intubation is found to be difficult after induction of general anaesthesia, may well be suitable for fibreoptic intubation, provided that the airway is easy to maintain and that not too many attempts at intubation have been undertaken, which tend to

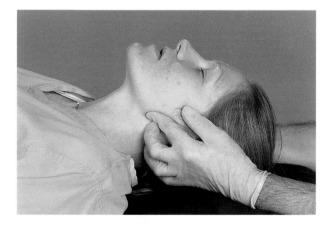

Fig. 5.3
Jaw thrust: note how the operator's fingers are placed correctly behind the angle of the mandible.

bloody the airway and create a lot of secretions.

It will be obvious to the experienced anaesthetist that at the end of general anaesthesia the trachea should on no account be extubated until the patient is capable of maintaining and protecting their airway.

MANAGEMENT OF EMERGENCY CASES

There is no doubt that fibreoptic intubation is a valuable aid in carefully selected emergency cases. Despite the effect of local anaesthesia on the protective reflexes of the upper airway, most practitioners would regard this as a technique of choice for the known, or suspected, difficult intubation in a patient with a full stomach. The safety of this technique has been confirmed in a large study. Fibreoptic intubation in pregnancy is best performed following the normal antacid regimen of H_2 (histamine type 2) blocker, such as ranitidine and 30 ml 0.3 molar sodium citrate antacid.

Patients with facial injury may sometimes be intubated fibreoptically, but when there is profuse airway bleeding an awake crico-thyroidotomy, tracheostomy or a retrograde wire are more appropriate techniques. Basal skull fractures preclude the nasal route, although a careful and experienced endoscopist could establish whether it is safe by first performing a nasoendoscopy.

Where there is complete airway obstruction a fibreoptic intubation should not be attempted.

PAEDIATRIC FIBREOPTIC INTUBATION

Age alone is not a barrier to this technique, but clearly there are caveats. The paediatric fibreoptic laryngoscopes range from 2.4 mm in diameter to adult size, depending on the size of the child, and it is possible to pass a 3-mm endotracheal tube over the smallest of these. However, instruments of this size are thin and floppy and do not form a really effective stylet. Children also do not take kindly to large, oddly dressed people putting strange objects in their airway, and although awake fibreoptic intubation is possible in children, more often than not the amount of sedation required makes general anaesthesia a safer bet.

One particularly useful technique for the paediatric fibreoptic intubator is the 'anterograde wire' technique. If a scope is too large to take an appropriately small endotracheal tube, then the available scope can be passed to the laryngeal inlet and a guidewire passed down the working channel of the scope and into the trachea. After the scope has been removed, the endotracheal tube can be railroaded over the wire. If the wire is considered too floppy for good railroading, a paediatric size exchange bougie, or wire stiffener, can be threaded over the wire and the endotracheal tube railroaded over it.

6

Complications of fibreoptic intubation

In this chapter most of the problems encountered during fibreoptic intubation will be described. The methods of prevention and treatment of the complications are also discussed.

THE WORST SCENARIO

Faced with a difficult and compromised airway the most important thing to remember is to avoid doing anything from the preparation of the patient to securing the endotracheal tube in position that could precipitate the loss of the airway. It is essential to have a back-up plan in case the airway is lost before it is secured. Be especially careful in the presence of tumour and oedema as they can change size rapidly when traumatised.

If the airway obstructs, apply the routine difficult airway manoeuvres; these should be known if a practitioner is performing any solo endoscopies.

Under general anaesthesia this may be simple muscular paralysis for laryngospasm, using a laryngeal mask airway, a bougie or a McCoy laryngoscope, to some form of tracheal access. If it is a difficult airway requiring an awake technique, it is wise if the airway is lost completely to have a quick look with a normal laryngoscope to see if intubation is possible. If it is not, then access to the airway must be achieved via the crico-thyroid membrane. Remember that there is an obstructed upper airway and therefore exhalation must occur via this route to avoid barotrauma. Patients in this situation quickly become uncontrollable and must be anaesthetised quickly and intravenously. Not only is this humane, but it will be nearly impossible to secure the airway with the patient fighting for life. Obviously, if the patient can be kept awake and breathing, this is best for survival; at least the patient may breathe if a hole appears anywhere leading to the lower airway.

When faced with a severely compromised airway, one of the best things to do is to have the local Ear, Nose and Throat specialist standing by the patient, scalpel in hand, and local anaesthetic with epinephrine already infiltrated over the proposed site of incision. It should be understood that the rapid creation of a hole in the trachea is what is required should things go wrong. A tracheostomy or endotracheal tube can be inserted rapidly, with or without the aid of a bougie; one can even pass the fibreoptic laryngoscope into the trachea and railroad a tube over this. Using the fibreoptic laryngoscope has the added advantage of being able to see that the trachea has been entered and that a false passage has not been made in the subcutaneous tissues. Oxygen can also be jetted into the trachea using the working channel of the scope, taking care to allow the gas to escape. There is no room for the definitive tracheostomy in this situation; it takes too long.

POOR VISION

Inexperience

This is the commonest cause for a poor endoscopic view. The secret of successful fibreoptic intubation rests in the ability to maintain a good view at all times by keeping the insertion tube in the midline and aiming for the centre of the airspace in front. Remember that if the patient is approached from the front, the up–down orientation of the endoscopic view is inverted; the inferior part of the image through the scope will actually be superior in the patient. Approaching the patient from behind in the first few attempts at fibreoptic intubation is best as this orientation problem is avoided (Figs. 6.1 and 6.2).

Any technique takes time and practice to learn and it is no different with fibreoptic intubation. Good instruction in the first instance, together with regular practice will ensure that failures are few. Evidence shows that when competent, the success rate in a well-prepared theatre patient is ~95–97%.

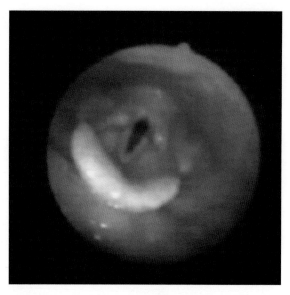

Fig. 6.2
Inverted view of the larynx obtained when performing an endoscopy from in front of the patient.

Obviously, the more difficult the anatomy, the higher the failure rate, even in the best hands. Awake nasal techniques are easier to perform and have a higher success rate than fibreoptic intubation performed under general anaesthesia or when using an oral approach.

Poorly focused eyepiece

Adjust the eyepiece focus ring while holding the tip of the instrument ~1–1.5 cm above some typescript. Try and keep the tip pointing straight at the object in focus.

Film over the lens

After several sterilisations, a thin film can develop over the lenses of the fibreoptic laryngoscope. Cleaning them with an alcohol wipe easily rectifies this problem.

Fogging

When fogging occurs, the view will appear misty and unclear and is known as a 'white out' (Fig. 6.3). This happens because the warm water from the airway condenses on the tip of the cold scope. Either dip the tip of the scope in some warm water (max 60°C) or hold it against a mucosal surface for ~30 s before use. Alternatively, a commercially available anti-fogging solution, a silicone solution or a weak soap solution can be used.

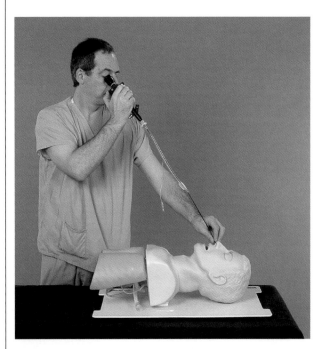

Fig. 6.1
Position taken when intubating from the front.

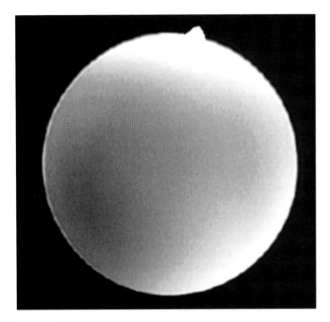

Fig. 6.3
Fogged image ('white out') with the carina vaguely visible.

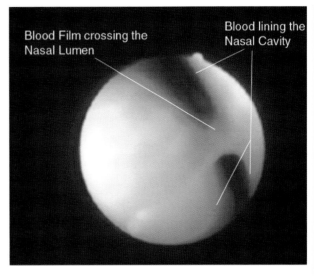

Fig. 6.4
With this amount of blood, it is difficult to maintain a clear view.

Secretions and blood

The upper airway secretes mucus and saliva, particularly when a foreign body stimulates it, or when certain pharmacological agents are used, such as the volatile agents and ketamine. Secretions or blood from the procedure or from trauma can totally obliterate the view (Figs. 6.4 and 6.5).

If there is a problem with secretions it may be possible to suck the offending material up the working channel of the fibreoptic laryngoscope; however, the secretions are often too tenacious to pass up such a small suction channel. A suction catheter can be passed down through the nose or mouth to suck out the pharynx, or some oxygen or saline can be flushed down the working channel of the scope in the hope that it clears the problem. Be aware that it has been known for gastric distension to occur when oxygen is insufflated down the working channel of a fibreoptic laryngoscope. If all the above fail, then remove the scope, clean it and try again.

The prophylactic use of an antisialagogue and sucking out the pharynx immediately before endoscopy will minimise the problems created by upper airway secretions and in the awake patient asking them to swallow can help.

Touching the mucosa

When the tip of the scope touches a mucosal surface it transilluminates the mucosa and vessels

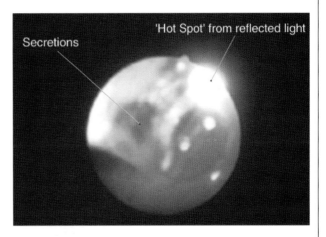

Fig. 6.5
Fibreoptic view degraded by secretions.

giving a 'red out' (Fig. 6.6). The first thing to do is to reverse the movement that brought the scope into contact with the mucosal surface. If this does not work pull the scope back a little. This should solve most problems in the upper airway. As a final resort, gently flex the tip of the scope in the opposite direction to which it is pointing, but be very careful not to force this movement as damage can occur to the mucosal surface. This may cause bleeding, which will just worsen the situation.

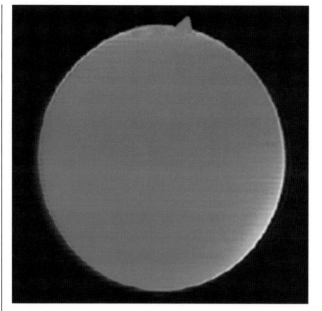

Fig. 6.6
'Red out' obtained when the tip of the scope touches a mucosal surface.

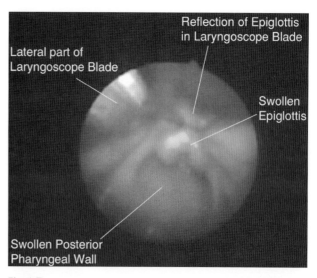

Fig. 6.7
A very swollen pharynx opened up by direct laryngoscopy to allow access for the fibreoptic laryngoscope.

Repetitive swallowing

Swallowing involves the movement of the larynx cranially towards the tip of the scope. When this is uncontrollable it is almost impossible to succeed with a fibreoptic intubation. In the awake patient swallowing can occur when the cuff of an airway situated in the nasopharynx is inflated in an attempt to stem the blood flow from an epistaxis (Fig. 6.9). Unfortunately there is no satisfactory solution to this problem if it occurs.

Abnormal anatomy

With abnormal anatomy it is especially important to aim for the centre of the open airway, as the usual landmarks are often missing. Just following the air space in front is sometimes all that is possible, trying to identify the laryngeal inlet as it is approached. If the air passage does not lead to the larynx then withdraw the laryngoscope until some normal anatomy or the airspace is seen, and try again.

The upper airway in the obese or in patients with sleep apnoea can close under general anaesthesia and intermittently in severe cases when awake. Try manoeuvres that will help to open the pharynx (see Chapter 7) including placing the tip of the fibreoptic laryngoscope beneath the epiglottis while lifting the epiglottis away from the posterior pharyngeal wall by performing a direct laryngoscopy (Fig. 6.7). It is possible to do this awake if the airway anaesthesia is good or if the situation becomes desperate.

BLEEDING

Up to one-quarter of nasal fibreoptic intubations cause some bleeding and bleeding can occur anywhere the fibreoptic laryngoscope, an endotracheal tube or a needle are passed. Most bleeding is inconsequential, but occasionally it can be so heavy that it is necessary to abandon the procedure, which will alter the management of the airway. Suction can be used to clear the view, but the blood usually re-accumulates (Fig. 6.8). One way to overcome the problem is to pass an endotracheal tube into the pharynx and then pass the scope through it. Using the endotracheal tube as a conduit

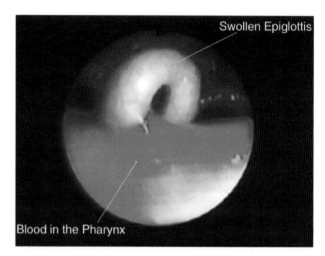

Fig. 6.8
Here it will be difficult to negotiate under the epiglottis without covering the tip of the insertion tube with blood.

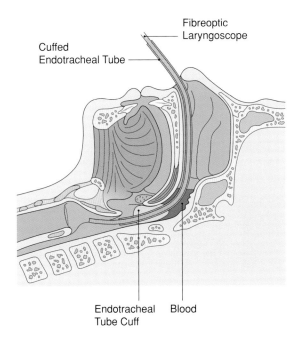

Fig. 6.9
Pulling the nasal tube back with the cuff partially inflated.

keeps the fibreoptic laryngoscope away from the posterior pharyngeal wall and the blood. Nasal intubation is more effective in this situation as the tube tends to sit nicely in the pharynx and usually points towards the larynx. The tube can also tamponade the bleeding if it is coming from the nose or the cuff can be blown up when it is in the nasopharynx and then pulled gently back until it occludes the bleeding nostril (Fig. 6.9). Be aware that in the awake patient this manoeuvre can cause uncontrollable swallowing.

Orally, try using a fibreoptic intubating airway.

Haematomas

Haematomas have been known to occur around the site of local anaesthetic injections. Most are harmless, but following a crico-thyroid stab they can compress the airway. The internal laryngeal and glossopharyngeal nerve blocks are less likely to do this in a patient with normal anatomy as the upper airway diameter in these positions is much greater.

It is wise to use a 'spray as you go' technique in a patient who is taking anticoagulants or who has a coagulopathy.

COUGHING

A crico-thyroid stab will usually cause coughing and is therefore best avoided in a patient with an

unstable cervical spine, or if the airway is severely compromised. If it happens during laryngoscopy, it indicates that there is inadequate anaesthesia, be it general or local. The problems can range from temporarily losing the view to total loss of vision, through to losing the airway altogether.

The following are ways to prevent or stop the coughing.

Improve anaesthesia

General anaesthesia can be taken to a deeper plane to suppress coughing or the muscles may be paralysed, if appropriate. If a local technique is being used, it is frequently inadequate anaesthesia of the laryngeal inlet or trachea that is the problem. A couple of good sprays of lidocaine down the working channel of the scope are usually sufficient to prevent further coughing. Sometimes coughing occurs when the spray hits the larynx, but this usually subsides. The same technique can also be applied during general anaesthesia.

Give opioids

Short-acting opioids, such as alfentanil, are very effective in obtunding the cough reflex, but always be aware that it is possible to lose a severely compromised airway with this technique. Respiratory depression may also occur, although this can be controlled by the administration of small doses of the opioid antagonist naloxone.

Give sedatives

Drugs such as the short-acting benzodiazipine, midazolam also suppress coughing. However, the use of midazolam may also result in the loss of the airway and respiratory depression.

Intravenous lidocaine

Intravenous lidocaine not only suppresses the cough reflex, but it also has the added advantage of suppressing any pressor response to the intubation.

A dose of up to 1 mg/kg may be used. However, it should be remembered that intravenous lidocaine should be avoided in patients with cardiac failure or hypovolaemia.

HAEMOGLOBIN DESATURATION

The following are the causes of haemoglobin oxygen desaturation directly related to fibreoptic intubation.

Hypostimulation

There is a tendency for desaturation to occur when breathing spontaneously under general anaesthesia during a fibreoptic intubation, as there is little stimulation of the patient for several minutes while the endoscopy takes place. This can result in respiratory depression. Increasing the inspired oxygen concentration helps to maintain an adequate saturation. Oxygen can also be administered by attaching an oxygen source, using a Luer lock connector, to the working channel of the fibreoptic laryngoscope; 2–3 litres/min (see glossary) at low pressure has been recommended. Always be aware that when insufflating oxygen there is a risk of barotrauma and gastric insufflation. Taking general anaesthesia to a lighter plane can also improve the situation, but be careful not to allow the return of the airway reflexes or to risk awareness.

Excessive use of suction

One cause of desaturation is the operation of the suction facility of the fibreoptic scope, which sucks gas away from the upper and lower airways. Therefore, avoid using the suction apparatus continuously.

Endobronchial intubation

Endobronchial intubation can be avoided by making sure that the carina can be seen as the insertion tube is withdrawn from the endotracheal tube and by making sure that the tip of the endotracheal tube is placed at the mid-tracheal position and not immediately above the carina.

Loss of the airway

Remember that with a difficult airway, desaturation may warn of impending or complete loss of the airway.

LARYNGOSPASM AND BRONCHOSPASM

Laryngospasm and bronchospasm occur due to inadequate anaesthesia, either local or general, and are mediated via stimulation of either the glossopharyngeal or vagus nerves.

If bronchospasm is the problem, treatment with a nebulised or intravenous bronchodilator should be started as soon as possible. Incremental doses of ketamine, up to 0.5 mg/kg, are very effective in producing bronchodilation. Ketamine has the least effect of all of the anaesthetic agents on upper airway tone, but remember that the patient may become dysphoric and salivate when it is used. Alternatively, small doses of epinephrine (25–50 μg) can be used. If the scope is already in the trachea and the bronchospasm is not too severe, then the endotracheal tube should be inserted and the bronchospasm treated at the earliest moment. Using a volatile agent once the airway is secure helps to relieve the spasm.

Laryngospasm should be treated by removal of the stimulus and by applying 100% oxygen with continuous positive airway pressure. If the patient is under general anaesthesia, then the depth of anaesthesia should be increased. If this fails, a depolarising muscle relaxant can be given provided it is thought that the lungs can be ventilated.

OESOPHAGEAL INTUBATION

There are several reasons why the oesophagus may be intubated inadvertently. The oesophagus may be mistaken for the trachea; hopefully this should not happen once an anaesthetist is competent at recognising normal, then abnormal anatomy through the fibreoptic laryngoscope. However, it can still occur after the tip of the laryngoscope has passed into the trachea. If the scope is not far into the trachea, railroading the endotracheal tube can cause

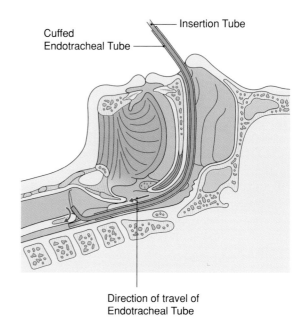

Fig. 6.10
Fibreoptic laryngoscope being pulled out of the larynx.

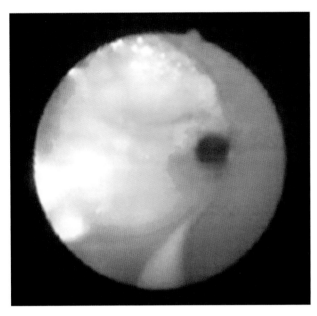

Fig. 6.11
Upper oesophageal sphincter as seen from the tip of an endotracheal tube.

the insertion tube to bend and flip out of the larynx and into the oesophagus, or nearby (Figs. 6.10 and 6.11). This is more likely to occur if the difference between the size of the endotracheal tube lumen and the insertion tube diameter is large, or if the insertion tube of the scope is very floppy. Swallowing during the procedure also increases the risk of oesophageal intubation.

Ways to minimise the risk of oesophageal intubation

Choose the right scope

Avoid using a scope with a very flexible insertion tube, such as a paediatric type, as these bend more during railroading of the endotracheal tube.

Use a flexible endotracheal tube

Flexible endotracheal tubes follow the line of the insertion tube more reliably during railroading. Either use an 'armoured' tube or an 'Intubating Laryngeal Mask' endotracheal tube (Fig. 6.12), or place a pre-formed type in warm water before endoscopy; this will make it flexible for a few minutes. Positioning the warmed tube into the upper airway and using it as a conduit for the fibreoptic scope keeps it warm and flexible.

Be far enough down the trachea

Ensure that the scope is at the mid-tracheal level before the endotracheal tube is railroaded (Fig. 6.13). Some authorities suggest that the tip of the scope should be placed further down the trachea, but one must always be aware of the risk of precipitating an untoward cardiac or respiratory reflex by stimulating un-anaesthetised trachea or carina. The best way to ensure correct positioning of the endotracheal tube is to continue observation

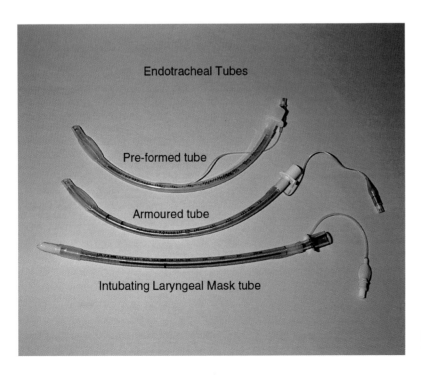

Endotracheal Tubes

Pre-formed tube

Armoured tube

Intubating Laryngeal Mask tube

Fig. 6.12
Three types of endotracheal tube.

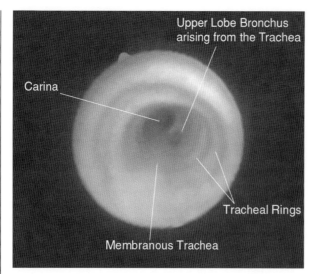

Fig. 6.13
Carina viewed from about mid-trachea. Remember that the trachea is only 10–12 cm long; note the abnormal origin of the upper lobe bronchus.

through the laryngoscope when railroading and to watch the endotracheal tube enter the trachea as it passes over the tip of the scope. The scope should then be passed to the end of the tube to observe the tracheal rings and carina and to adjust the position of the endotracheal tube as necessary. Make sure that the endotracheal tube is far enough down the trachea and not in the hypolarynx, where the cuff may damage the larynx and cause a recurrent laryngeal nerve palsy.

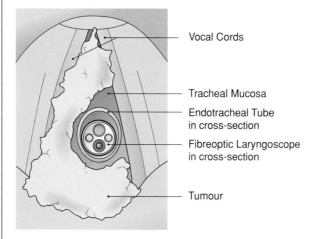

Fig. 6.14
How a fibreoptic laryngoscope can obliterate a small airway leaving little room for exhaled gas to escape.

BAROTRAUMA

Pneumothoraces can occur if the lower airway pressure rises excessively. This can occur if the upper airway anatomy is a tight fit around the fibreoptic laryngoscope such that the expiratory gas flow is impeded when oxygen is insufflated down the working channel of the scope. Be especially careful after the endotracheal tube has been railroaded over the insertion tube into the trachea, when the insertion tube is a tight fit into the endotracheal tube (Fig. 6.14). Oxygen insufflation down the working channel, when both the endotracheal tube is inside the trachea and the scope is still inside the tube, can cause a high-pressure surge below the larynx because there is little escape for the oxygen. This situation is very dangerous.

CARDIOVASCULAR RESPONSES

Hypertensive response

A hypertensive response seems to occur under general anaesthesia, comparable with that seen during a normal intubation, but there seems to be less of a response with a good local anaesthetic technique. Under general anaesthesia deepen the plane of anaesthesia or use an opioid. When using a local anaesthetic technique, this response, if deemed potentially harmful, can be treated by any of the drugs normally used to lower blood pressure acutely, provided that the drugs do not relax the airway or impair ventilation.

Hypotension

Hypotension can be a problem under general anaesthesia and occurs because there is little stimulation for several minutes. Either lighten the plane of anaesthesia, if this is possible, or use fluids and vasopressors to restore an adequate blood pressure.

Arrhythmias

Stimulation of the region innervated by the internal laryngeal or the recurrent laryngeal nerves can cause brady- as well as tachyarrhythmias and there is also a naso-cardiac reflex in which a bradycardia results from nasal stimulation. Good anaesthesia and analgesia should minimise this problem. If feasible, remove the stimulus causing the arrhythmia and try carotid sinus massage, which may help control a tachycardia temporarily. If these manoeuvres do not help, then pharmacological control of the arrhythmia is required.

PAIN AND AWARENESS

Because of the stimulation that occurs when the endotracheal tube is railroaded through the larynx, the patient will require as much anaesthetic agent and opioid to suppress awareness as during a normal intubation under general anaesthesia. Under local anaesthesia, with good pre-operative counselling, good communication between the operator and patient, and a good local anaesthetic technique, the incidence of unpleasant recall should be small. The majority of patients will consent to being intubated in a similar fashion again. Sedatives and opioids lower the incidence of unpleasant or painful experience, but the pros and cons of sedation/analgesia must be balanced against the condition of the airway. Once the airway is secure, a benzodiazipine may help in minimising recall.

Always remember that agitation may be due to hypoxaemia and may be unrelated to the chosen technique.

REGURGITATION

Theory suggests that good local anaesthesia can abolish the upper airway reflexes sufficiently to allow aspiration of gastric contents, but this has never been shown to be a problem in practice. However, if a patient is at high risk of regurgitation, then it is prudent, if time allows, for full starvation and premedication with an H$_2$ (histamine type 2) antagonist such as ranitidine, a prokinetic such as metoclopramide and 30 ml 0.3 molar sodium citrate antacid just before endoscopy. It is also worthwhile to consider performing the intubation in the sitting position.

Under general anaesthesia the normal rules apply, and fibreoptic intubation can be performed with cricoid pressure. However, only an experienced endoscopist should do this as the time available to secure the airway will be limited and cricoid pressure can distort the anatomy.

Use of oxygen insufflation via the fibreoptic working channel can distend the stomach, which increases the risk of regurgitation.

VOMITING

The vomiting reflex can occur in response to fibreoptic endoscopy. Better local anaesthesia and sedation can help. Vomiting does not occur under general anaesthesia.

GASTRIC DISTENSION AND RUPTURE

Distension of the stomach has been reported when oxygen has been delivered to the upper airway via the working channel of the fibreoptic laryngoscope or via pharyngeal catheters. It seems important to avoid using high gas pressure and high flows, and to avoid insufflation when the scope is in, or close to, the upper oesophagus. Gastric rupture has been reported.

POST-EXTUBATION OBSTRUCTION

The partially obstructed airway is at particular risk of post-extubation obstruction, so meticulous observation is essential. Some patients require a prolonged period of intubation until the obstructing pathology resolves or is dealt with definitively, and these patients are best looked after in an Intensive Care Unit. If stridor develops after extubation, a helium and oxygen mixture improves gas flow past the obstruction, which allows more time to treat the problem definitively.

EQUIPMENT PROBLEMS

Lighting

Light failure can occur during a fibreoptic laryngoscopy. This can be due to a simple disconnection of the umbilical from the light source, a light source failure or the battery of a portable scope running out. The problem can be dealt with by using another fibreoptic system or the procedure postponed until another day. If it is essential to proceed, then it may be necessary to secure the airway in a different manner.

Foreign bodies

In theory, pieces of the fibreoptic laryngoscope can be lost in the upper airway, however it is more likely that pieces or whole parts of the ancillary equipment may become disconnected and lodge in the airway, such as segments of the endoscopy mask diaphragm or the tip of the local anaesthetic spray.

7

Tricks, tips and techniques

OPENING THE PHARYNGEAL AIRWAY

FAILURE TO RAILROAD THE ENDOTRACHEAL TUBE

CANNOT ADVANCE/RETRACT THE FIBREOPTIC LARYNGOSCOPE

USE OF THE LARYNGEAL MASK AIRWAY

RETROGRADE WIRE TECHNIQUE

NON RAILROAD TECHNIQUE

TRANSILLUMINATION

OPENING THE PHARYNGEAL AIRWAY

There are several manoeuvres that can open the upper airway if it is small or collapses. They can lift the base of the tongue, clear the epiglottis from a posterior position and open the pharynx, which will make any fibreoptic intubation a lot easier.

Jaw thrust

A finger, or knuckle, should be placed behind the angle of the jaw bilaterally and the whole mandible displaced anteriorly (Fig. 5.3).

Anterior tongue traction

Anterior tongue traction can be applied by grasping the tongue with some gauze, or non-traumatic Duval's forceps (e.g. lung forceps), and then pulling the tongue forwards and out of the mouth (Fig. 7.1). Not only is the tongue immobilised and the supraglottic tissues lifted and the pharynx opened, but it also has the effect of inhibiting swallowing and biting. However, do not pull the tongue over the teeth as it is easily lacerated. This is also a useful manoeuvre to use if the tongue tries to manipulate the insertion tube.

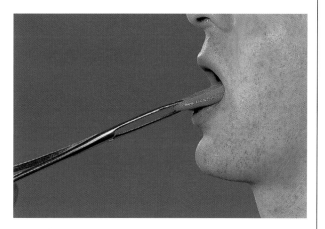

Fig. 7.1
Anterior tongue traction using Duval's forceps.

Laryngeal lift

The larynx can be elevated manually by grasping the thyroid cartilage on the anterior neck and gently lifting. It is best if this is not done to the awake patient because it is very uncomfortable (Fig. 7.2).

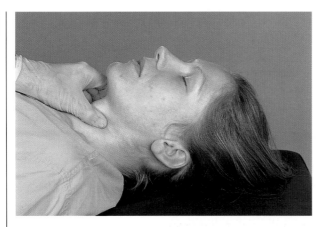

Fig. 7.2
Laryngeal lift.

Change patient position

In the awake patient, sitting them up helps open the pharynx. Sometimes the patient will present in the position in which it is easiest for them to breathe. In facial trauma, for instance, patients will sit forward and move their position so that any loose tissue falls away from the upper airway. This will usually be the best position in which to try and intubate the trachea. It is common to suffer orientation problems in unusual positions, so think before starting which way will be up when endoscopy has commenced.

Normal laryngoscopy

Getting a second operator to perform a normal laryngoscopy at the same time as a fibreoptic intubation is attempted is sometimes helpful, especially if the soft tissues of the upper airway are swollen (Fig. 6.7). This can be done under local anaesthesia if the upper airway is well anaesthetised, or if the situation becomes desperate.

Continuous positive airway pressure – a warning

It has been said that insufflating oxygen or applying nasal CPAP can aid the opening of the pharynx. However, high pressure can be generated in the upper airway, which can cause distension of the stomach, which may precipitate the regurgitation of gastric contents or rupture of the stomach.

FAILURE TO RAILROAD THE ENDOTRACHEAL TUBE

It is always a good feeling when the tip of the fibreoptic laryngoscope passes through the larynx, especially if the airway has been difficult. Unfortunately, it is still possible to fail to intubate the trachea and this can have disastrous consequences if if it is a severely compromised airway.

There are several reasons why there may be problems with railroading.

The tube may be too large to pass through the nostril

This can occur if the nostril has not been pre-sized before mounting the endotracheal tube on to the scope. As mentioned before, this can be avoided if both nasal passages are pre-inspected with the endoscope before performing the definitive laryngoscopy or if an endotracheal tube is passed through the nose and into the pharynx before endoscopy.

Anatomical hang-ups

The commonest cause of an endotracheal tube not passing easily into the trachea is when the tip of the tube catches on either the epiglottis or another part of the laryngeal inlet, usually the right arytenoid (Fig. 7.3). It has also been known for bony abnormalities, such as an osteophyte or deformed rheumatoid vertebra, to impinge on the pharynx and impede the passage of the endotracheal tube. It is useful to note anything such as this during the endoscopy so that the endotracheal tube can be manipulated appropriately during railroading.

'Hanging up' occurs in ~25% of cases and there are several ways to minimise this problem.

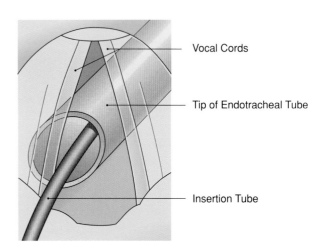

Vocal Cords

Tip of Endotracheal Tube

Insertion Tube

Fig. 7.3
Tip of the endotracheal tube caught in the laryngeal sinus (ventricle). However, the commonest place to hang-up is on the arytenoid cartilages.

How to combat 'hanging-up'

There are certain things that the anaesthetist can do to minimise the risk of the endotracheal tube from hanging-up and there are certain manoeuvres that can correct the problem once it has arisen.

How to prevent hanging-up of the endotracheal tube

Use the nasal approach

Hanging-up occurs less frequently with a nasal approach. Oral intubation techniques suffer from difficulties in railroading the endotracheal tube in 20–35% of cases, whereas with a nasal approach this can be as low as 6%.

Use the correct endotracheal tube

A flexible, armoured or a conical tipped endotracheal tube will hang-up on fewer occasions than the more rigid endotracheal tubes or those with a prominent bevel (Fig. 7.4). Warming a normal pre-formed endotracheal tube in water makes it flexible for a few minutes and also helps minimise any trauma during its passage past the nasal turbinates. The Intubating Laryngeal Mask endotracheal tube hangs-up less frequently than normal or armoured tubes.

Match the insertion tube and endotracheal sizes

If there is too large a gap between the outside diameter of the insertion tube and the inside diameter of the endotracheal tube, the incidence of 'hanging-up' is increased. This occurs because it is easier for the tip of the endotracheal tube to impinge upon the larynx. Therefore, make this gap as small as possible while still allowing the endotracheal tube to slide over the insertion tube. A larger scope or a smaller tube can be used (Figs 7.5 and 7.6). Alternatively, fit a small endotracheal tube inside one which is 2.5 mm larger, and remove the smaller inner tube once intubation has been completed. Make sure that the tip of the smaller tube protrudes through the larger by ~2–3 cm, as this smoothes out the profile of the advancing tube system. The connector will have to be removed from the outer endotracheal tube and be replaced once it has been successfully railroaded. Therefore, it is wise to make sure that the connector is easy to replace before beginning the procedure.

When the tube system is in the trachea, advance the outer tube over the inner, withdraw the fibreoptic laryngoscope and replace the connector. Because of the increased stiffness of the endotracheal tube system, this technique may be more prone to causing the scope to flip out of the trachea, so be careful.

When using an oral technique, it is possible to cut the outer tube to length and leave the inner at full length, so ensuring access to the top end of both endotracheal tubes (Fig. 7.7). With an uncut tube for a nasal intubation, it may be found that the top end of the inner endotracheal tube will need to sit inside the outer tube. If this is the case, then it is prudent to tie a strong silk thread to the top of the smaller inner tube, so that it can be stabilised when the larger endotracheal tube is railroaded into the trachea.

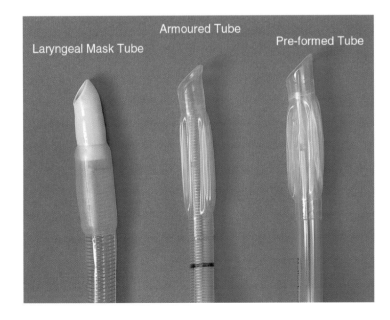

Laryngeal Mask Tube

Armoured Tube

Pre-formed Tube

Fig. 7.4
Tips of three endotracheal tubes. The frequency of hanging-up increases from left to right.

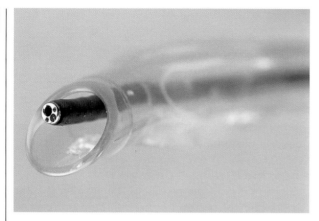

Fig. 7.5
Note the large bevel that can catch onto the larynx.

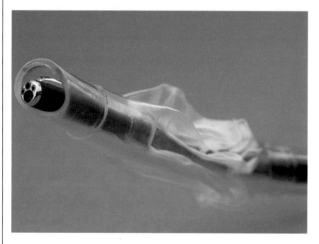

Fig. 7.6
Note the small gap between the insertion and endotracheal tubes. This helps minimise the risk of hanging-up.

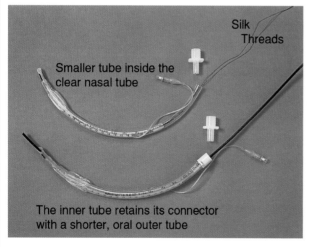

Silk
Threads

Smaller tube inside the
clear nasal tube

The inner tube retains its connector
with a shorter, oral outer tube

Fig. 7.7
Top tube system with a silk tie attached to the inner endotracheal tube for nasal intubation. In the lower set of tubes the outer tube has been cut to the length required for an oral intubation.

Deep inhalation

In the conscious patient, ask them to take a deep inspiration at the time of railroading the endotracheal tube. This lifts the uvula, opens the pharynx and opens the vocal cords widely, allowing an easier passage for the endotracheal tube.

Techniques to try if 'hanging-up' occurs

If the endotracheal tube 'hangs-up' during railroading, there are several manoeuvres that can be tried to overcome the problem. Never force the tube.

Pull back and twist

Pull the endotracheal tube back 1 or 2 cm, rotate it through 90° anticlockwise and try again. If it still hangs-up, then rotate it back to its original position and then 90° in the opposite direction before trying to advance it once more. Avoid twisting without first withdrawing the tube because this is likely to traumatise the larynx. Try inserting the endotracheal tube with the bevel facing inferiorly from the outset.

Head and neck manoeuvres

Useful techniques include jaw thrust (or removing it if it is already applied), flexion or extension of the head and neck, cricoid pressure, or, sometimes better, thyroid cartilage pressure (or removing pressure if they are already applied). A laryngeal lift or anterior tongue traction can also be tried.

Normal laryngoscopy

Lifting the tongue and soft tissues with a normal laryngoscope, as in a direct laryngoscopy, opens the upper airway and can make railroading easier.

Digital manipulation

Gentle digital manipulation of the insertion tube sometimes moves the tube past the obstruction.

Endotracheal tube sticking

If the insertion tube and the inside of the endotracheal tube are too snug a fit, or if the lubrication has been forgotten or has dried out, railroading can be difficult due to friction between the insertion and endotracheal tubes. On other occasions a loop of insertion tube can form in the upper airway preventing railroading, so ensure that the insertion tube is reasonably straight before advancing the endotracheal tube over it (Fig. 7.8). This is more likely to occur with a thin, floppy insertion tube.

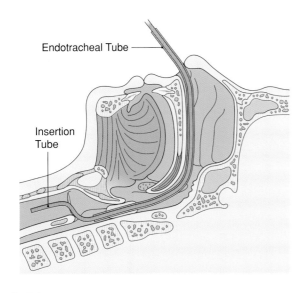

Fig. 7.8
Endotracheal tube hanging down in the pharynx after it has followed a loop of insertion tube to that position.

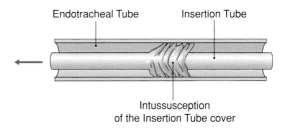

Fig. 7.9
How an intussusception of the outer cover of the fibreoptic laryngoscope can prevent withdrawal of the scope from the endotracheal tube.

CANNOT ADVANCE/RETRACT THE FIBREOPTIC LARYNGOSCOPE

Difficulty in advancing or retracting the fibreoptic laryngoscope, can be due to the lubrication drying out. It has also been known for the outer cover of the fibreoptic laryngoscope to intussuscept over the insertion tube and stick in the endotracheal tube when withdrawing the scope (Fig. 7.9).

Advancement as well as withdrawal can be difficult if the insertion tube has inadvertently passed through the Murphy's eye (see glossary) at the tip of the endotracheal tube when loading it on to the scope (Fig. 7.10). A quick check before the endoscopy will prevent this from happening. If the endotracheal tube has initially been placed in the upper airway, then pass the scope through the tube under direct vision and follow the radio-opaque blue line, which will avoid going through the Murphy's eye. In any of these situations the golden rule is not to force the instrument, as it is easy to inflict serious damage to the insertion tube. At worst, the laryngoscope and endotracheal tube will have to be withdrawn and the procedure repeated.

USE OF THE LARYNGEAL MASK AIRWAY

A Laryngeal Mask Airway (LMA) can guide the fibreoptic laryngoscope to the laryngeal inlet. When the fibreoptic laryngoscope has entered the trachea an endotracheal tube can be railroaded over the scope and through the LMA (see Appendix III for tube sizes). Removal of the aperture bars of a standard LMA can make the railroading easier (Fig. 7.11).

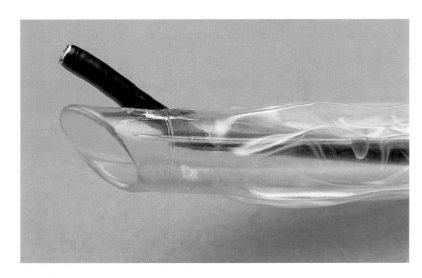

Fig. 7.10
Tip of an insertion tube which has passed through the 'Murphy's eye' of the endotracheal tube.

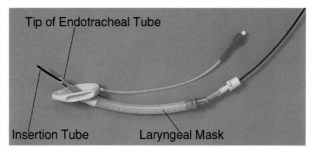

Tip of Endotracheal Tube

Insertion Tube   Laryngeal Mask

Fig. 7.11
Use of the laryngeal mask as a conduit for the fibreoptic
laryngoscope and endotracheal tube.

Once the trachea has been intubated, the LMA-
endotracheal tube unit can be left *in-situ* (Fig. 7.12),
or the LMA can be removed over the endotracheal
tube. The latter usually requires removal of the
endotracheal tube connector and the use of a rod to
keep a downward pressure on the end of the
endotracheal tube to prevent it from being pulled
out by the LMA as it is removed. Alternatively, a
guidewire can be passed through the working
channel of the scope and into the trachea, and the
scope and LMA removed. The wire can then be
used to pass the fibreoptic laryngoscope back
into the trachea and the tube railroaded as normal,
or a wire stiffener or exchange bougie can be passed
over the wire and the endotracheal tube railroaded
over this. Insertion of a large endotracheal tube
usually involves this two-stage procedure, unless
an 'intubating LMA' is available, which
accommodates an 8-mm endotracheal tube (Fig.
7.13).

Remember that the LMA can be attached to
an angle piece, which can then be connected to
the anaesthetic delivery circuit to allow
ventilation of the lungs while performing the
endoscopy via the nasal route. Once the tip of
the scope is above the cuff of the LMA, the LMA
can be removed with the cuff deflated and the
endoscopic intubation continued. This technique
is useful for teaching novices to minimise the
period of apnoea.

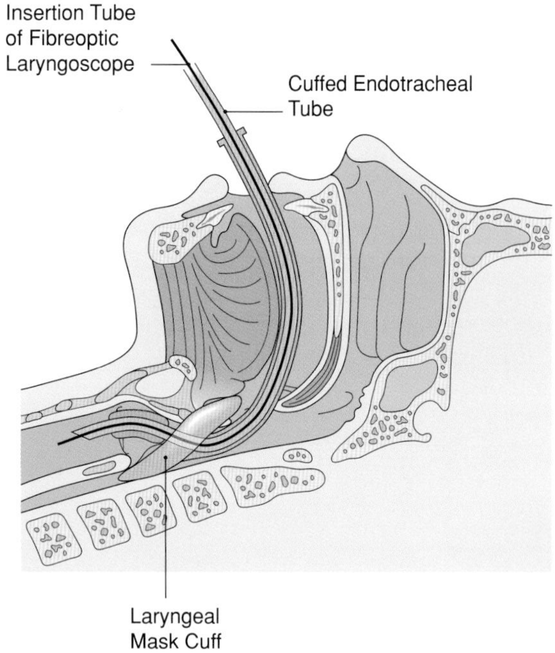

Insertion Tube
of Fibreoptic
Laryngoscope

Cuffed Endotracheal
Tube

Laryngeal
Mask Cuff

Fig. 7.12
Use of the laryngeal mask as a conduit for the fibreoptic
laryngoscope and endotracheal tube.

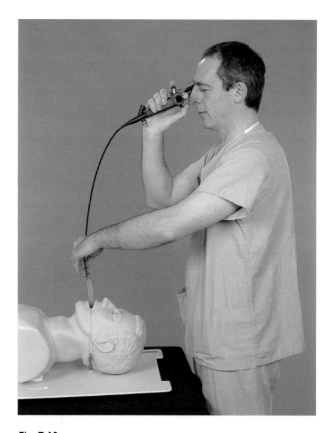

Fig. 7.13
Fibreoptic endoscopy utilising a laryngeal mask. With no
endotracheal tube loaded on to the fibreoptic laryngoscope, the
operator would have to pass a guidewire through the working
channel of the scope and railroad over this.

RETROGRADE WIRE TECHNIQUE

This is a good technique to use if bleeding above the larynx is making intubation difficult.

Guidewire

If a guidewire can be placed in a retrograde fashion from the trachea, through the larynx, to the nose or mouth, then the fibreoptic laryngoscope can be passed over the wire and into the trachea using the scope's working channel. 'Retrograde wire kits' are now available, but cardiac catheter wires or epidural catheters can be utilised instead. A 'J'-tipped wire is recommended as it causes less damage to the airway mucosa or a tumourous mass (Fig. 7.14).

Conduit

Before the guidewire can be passed into the trachea, the anaesthetist must first place a channel through the anterior neck and into the trachea through which the wire will travel. Ready-made kits are available for this, but a Tuohy needle or intravenous cannula are commonly used; check that the wire can pass through the cannula before embarking on the technique. The crico-thyroid or crico-tracheal

membranes are the points usually used for the portal of entry; the crico-tracheal membrane has the advantage that it is further down the airway, which allows the scope, or endotracheal tube, to pass further into the trachea before the guidewire needs to be removed. It also avoids the crico-thyroid arteries that cross the crico-thyroid membrane.

Technique

The patient's head and neck need to be extended and the tissues overlying the crico-thyroid or crico-tracheal membrane anaesthetised; lidocaine with epinephrine (1:200,000 – see glossary) is usually the most appropriate choice for infiltration as bleeding has to be minimal in this position. Application of local anaesthetic to the tracheal mucosa can be achieved using a crico-thyroid stab. The cannula is then advanced into the trachea in a perpendicular fashion. Once air is aspirated (putting some saline in the syringe shows the air bubbles), advance the conduit in a cranial direction. Preferably only a blunt and flexible conduit should be advanced into the trachea. Be very wary of puncturing the posterior tracheal wall; behind it lie some large vessels and the oesophagus — mediastinitis and severe haemorrhage can result. Therefore, it is prudent not to advance any type of needle very far into the trachea.

Advancing the guidewire

Hold the cannula tightly where it passes through the skin and gently pass the guidewire through it, into the trachea and up through the larynx. The wire can then be advanced through the mouth using Magill forceps (Fig. 7.15). To pass the wire nasally, place an endotracheal tube into the pharynx via the nose and then guide the wire through this. As an alternative, pass the wire through the mouth and tie it to a suction catheter that has been passed through the nose and out of the mouth. The suction catheter can then be used to pull the wire back through the nose.

Railroading

Before railroading anything over the wire, clamp it at the point where it enters the skin of the neck. This will make sure that the wire does not become dislodged. The fibreoptic laryngoscope can then be passed over the guidewire (Fig. 7.16). Avoid manipulating the tip of the scope once the wire is inside the working channel as this can cause damage to the insertion tube. Some difficulty may be

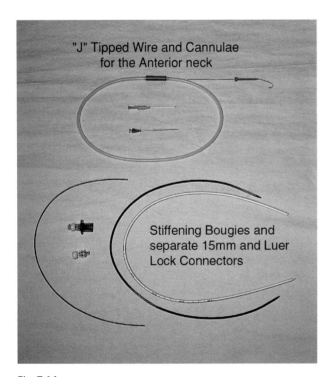

"J" Tipped Wire and Cannulae for the Anterior neck

Stiffening Bougies and separate 15mm and Luer Lock Connectors

Fig. 7.14
Retrograde wire kit, with stiffening bougies to go over the wire before railroading an endotracheal tube.

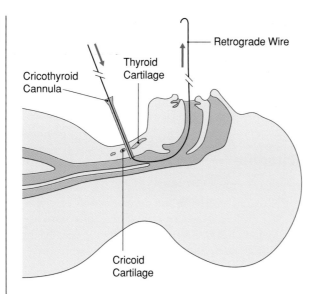

Fig. 7.15
A 'J' wire, which has been passed in a retrograde fashion through the crico-thyroid cannula.

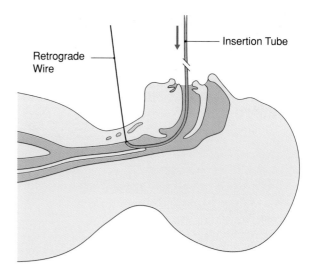

Fig. 7.16
The insertion tube has been passed over the retrograde wire as far as the entry point in the trachea.

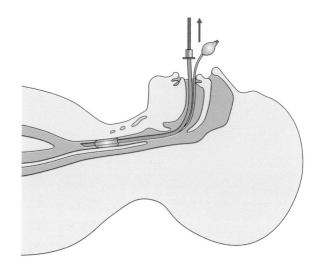

Fig. 7.17
The endotracheal tube has been fully railroaded into the trachea over the fibreoptic laryngoscope.

encountered once the scope has reached the point where the guidewire enters the trachea. This is a very short distance from the vocal cords and, after removal of the guidewire, it is possible for the insertion tube to flip out of the larynx. By using the fibreoptic laryngoscope the withdrawal of the guidewire can be visualised and the scope can then be passed further into the trachea prior to railroading the endotracheal tube (Fig. 7.17). A good guide to the scope remaining in the correct position is the bright midline anterior transillumination seen on the neck and visualisation of the tracheal rings. Avoid going right up to the mucosa with the scope, because this makes it impossible to see the wire being removed.

If railroading over the guidewire is chosen, be sure not to pull the wire too tight or the larynx may be 'cheese-wired'. Alternatively, another sheath, such as a cardiac catheter or an exchange bougie, can be threaded over the wire to decrease its flexibility before railroading the endotracheal tube into the trachea.

When the guidewire is removed it is best to pull it through the larynx and out of the nose or mouth. This helps prevent infection at the site where the wire has entered the trachea as only clean wire will have passed through that region, which is not the case if the wire is pulled back through the neck.

Morbidly obese patients or those with pre-tracheal masses are not good candidates for this technique due to the loss of normal landmarks. The use of the technique is also questionable in patients with a laryngeal tumour.

The presence of an infraglottic tumour contraindicates the use of the technique.

NON-RAILROAD TECHNIQUE

The tip of the fibreoptic laryngoscope can be placed just inside the tip of the endotracheal tube and the scope can be used to observe as the tube is manipulated through the larynx. Another way is to pass the scope through one nostril and the endotracheal tube down the other, so that the positioning of the endotracheal tube can be observed. This technique is useful when the endotracheal tube is too small to fit over the fibreoptic laryngoscope or if there are problems with repeated hanging-up during railroading.

TRANSILLUMINATION

If the fibreoptic endoscopist becomes lost because of difficult airway anatomy, he should look at the anterior neck for the light from the tip of the scope. A dark light suggests that it is very posterior, or in the oesophagus.

8

Care and maintenance

STORAGE

PRE-USE CHECKS

HANDLING OF THE FIBREOPTIC LARYNGOSCOPE

OTHER EQUIPMENT

LUBRICATION

CLEANING AND STERILISATION

SERVICING AND REPAIR

Due to the cost of fibreoptic instruments there is usually a limited number available in any one department. Therefore, teaching programmes should always include a section on care and maintenance of the instrument so that they remain functional for as long as possible. In addition, the inexperienced practitioner should be discouraged from using the fibreoptic laryngoscope until properly trained in the care and correct handling of the instrument.

STORAGE

When transporting the fibreoptic laryngoscope around the hospital, it should be kept in its carrying case, which will maintain it in the best possible position within a confined space and will prevent accidental damage.

When it comes to transportation by air, ensure that the ethylene oxide (ETO) venting cap is attached to the scope. This allows the pressure inside the scope to remain in equilibrium with the atmospheric pressure. If this is not done, it is possible for the cover of the scope to rupture during the flight (Fig. 8.1).

At all other times, it is best if the scope can hang within a straight container or cupboard to minimise the stress on the fibreoptic bundles and control wires. It is also best to avoid areas with high humidity and temperatures (inside a closed container), which promote bacterial and fungal growth. Sunlight can also damage the flexible cover of the scope, while X-rays (see glossary) can cause the fibreoptic bundles to change to a yellow colour.

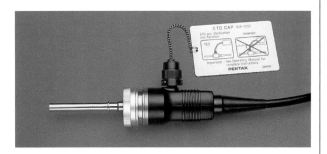

Fig. 8.1
If the scope is of the non-portable type, the attachment position for the ethylene oxide cap will be on the end of the umbilical. If it is a portable scope, it will be on the control body.

PRE-USE CHECKS

Disinfection and sterilisation

Before use, the anaesthetist should check to make sure that the scope has been leak-tested and sterilised (see below).

Movements

Prior to use, the fibreoptic laryngoscope should be checked to ensure that the control lever is operable in both directions and that the tip moves in harmony with it.

Patency of working channel

To test the patency of the working channel, inject saline or water down it (Fig. 8.2).

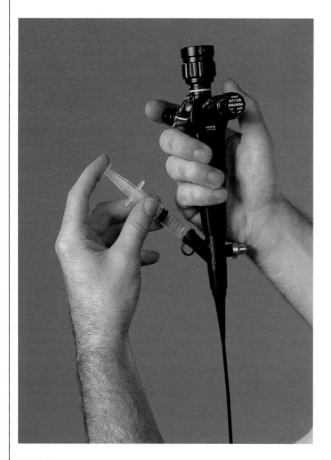

Fig. 8.2
Injecting saline down the working channel of a portable scope.

HANDLING OF THE FIBREOPTIC LARYNGOSCOPE

If it is appreciated that each individual fibre in the image transmitting fibreoptic bundle is only 6–10 µm in diameter and those of the light bundles ~10–15 µm in diameter, and that the whole system is contained within a thin plastic polymer sheath, then it is understandable how little force is necessary to damage a fibreoptic laryngoscope. Repairs usually run in the order of hundreds and sometimes thousands of pounds.

Fibreoptic trolley

When performing a fibreoptic intubation, there should be a trolley or cart specifically for the scope, light source and ancillary equipment. The trolley should allow the scope to be laid flat with no sharp bending of the insertion tube and umbilical. It should also be large enough so that no part of the scope protrudes over its sides. A sterile towel should cover the trolley to prevent scratching the outer cover of the scope and a second towel should be used to cover the instrument before use.

Manoeuvres to avoid

The following are manoeuvres that can cause damage to the fibreoptic laryngoscope, when performed with force:

- Axial twisting
- Bending or curling
- Tip flexion and extension – never do this manually as a control wire can break
- Railroading of the endotracheal tube – this can also cause damage to the insertion tube, especially if the tip is flexed or if the insertion tube is bent at an acute angle. Good lubrication minimises the risk of damage from this procedure
- Insertion/withdrawal – a fibreoptic laryngoscope that is stuck in the endotracheal tube should be removed with the tube *in-situ*. In addition, trying to insert or withdraw the instrument with the tip flexed or extended can damage the scope

Biting

A firm bite onto the insertion tube can completely destroy the fibreoptic bundles of a scope. Therefore, some form of bite block, such as an oral fibreoptic-intubating airway, should be used when performing an awake oral fibreoptic intubation.

OTHER EQUIPMENT

Light source

The light source should be checked to make sure that it works and that the scope fits the light source. If a portable scope is being used, make sure there are spare batteries to hand.

Ancillary equipment

Ensure that the fibreoptic laryngoscopy trolley is equipped with all the drugs and aids that may be required during an endoscopy and intubation.

A pre-operative check of the equipment may not be possible if there is an emergency difficult airway to deal with. Therefore, a system of regular checks (by a designated person) should be organised. Keeping a record of these checks is useful should it ever become necessary to prove that the equipment is maintained.

The following items should be available on a fibreoptic intubating trolley:

- Airways – oral and nasal
- Batteries for a portable scope – plus a spare set
- Bougies – a full range
- Crico-thyroidotomy kit
- Duval's forceps (lung) – for anterior tongue traction
- Endotracheal tubes – a full range
- Intubation or exchange catheter

- Krause's forceps
- Laryngeal masks – a full range
- Laryngoscope handles and blades – two handles and a range of blades, including a McCoy and a Polio
- Lidocaine and aqueous gel
- Lidocaine – 1–4%
- Local anaesthetic with epinephrine (1:200,000)
- Magill forceps
- Needles, syringes, intravenous cannulae and swabs
- Oral fibreoptic intubating airways
- Pharyngeal catheters/nasal cannulae/nasal cushions – for delivery of oxygen to the awake subject
- Retrograde wire kit
- Sterile gloves
- Suction catheters
- Sutures
- Swabs on sticks – to apply the local anaesthetic to the nose
- Vasoconstrictors for the nose – cocaine/xylometazoline/ephedrine

Any drugs necessary for a general anaesthetic should also be available at the time of intubation.

If a fibreoptic intubation is to be performed on a patient whose airway is compromised, in addition to the above, it is prudent to have a high-pressure oxygen injector available, such as a Sanders' injector, in case a crico-thyroid airway is required. The means by which to connect the airway to the injector should also be available and checked to ensure that it will fit the chosen airway (Fig. 8.3).

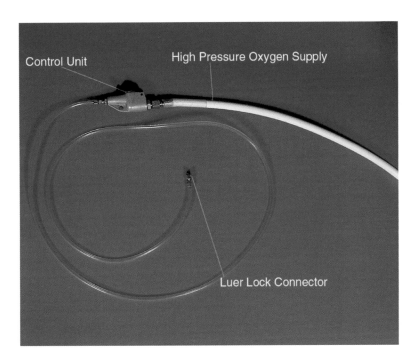

Fig. 8.3
Sanders' injector.

| ## LUBRICATION

Before use, the insertion tube should be smeared with a water-soluble lubricant, either aqueous or lidocaine gel. Lidocaine gel seems to dry more slowly than the aqueous variety and for this reason it is more useful, but avoid getting any on the lenses of the scope as this severely affects the image quality. Never use a petroleum-based lubricant as it can damage the outer flexible cover of the insertion tube.

Ideally, the scope should be wiped over with silicone oil every week. This helps to keep the flexible outer cover supple, gives some protection from corrosive elements, keeps the scope looking as new and lubricates the moving parts. The oil should be kept away from any electrical contacts.

CLEANING AND STERILISATION

Before cleaning the fibreoptic laryngoscope, check for any damage, especially to the outer protective plastic cover. Look especially at the distal 'bending rubber' covering the tip of the insertion tube and at the point where the insertion tube is joined to the control body (root brace seal). These areas are the most vulnerable parts of the scope. If there is any damage to the scope, just clean the debris from it. Be especially concerned if there is unexplained fogging of the lens during an endoscopy, as this may indicate that the integrity of the working channel has been disrupted. Washing or sterilisation in this situation will severely damage the instrument.

If there are concerns about the integrity of the fibreoptic laryngoscope, then it should be returned to the manufacturer for assessment.

Cleaning

All scopes should be cleaned after use. Initially, they should be wiped gently with a soft non-abrasive damp cloth. The submersible parts can then be washed in water or a weak soap solution. Note: all modern scopes are fully immersible (since 985). If in doubt, check with the manufacturer.

Usually instruments come with brushes to clean the working channel of the scope. These should be inserted from the top of the scope and not from the tip of the insertion tube (Fig. 8.4).

After using the brushes, flush saline and then blow air down the working channel to remove any debris left behind. Now dismantle the suction and injection port assemblies and clean them. After this test the scope for leaks.

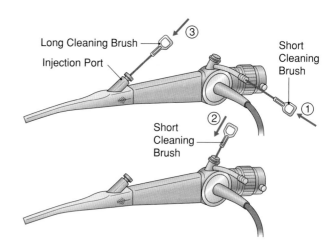

Fig. 8.4
Some systems use two brushes. The short brush pushes debris down to the injection port; the long brush cleans from this port to the end of the working channel.

Leak testing

Most hospitals have a policy stating that instruments such as the fibreoptic laryngoscope should be sterilised before use, but check first to see that the scope has been leak-tested. Ingress of any fluid through a hole or tear in the outer cover can degrade, or at worst destroy, the function of the fibreoptic bundles and the repair will involve the replacement of the insertion tube. Small tears can harbour body fluids and these can transmit infection from one patient to another. Therefore, testing for small and large holes in the cover is essential before use or sterilisation and involves a dry and a wet stage.

Dry testing

In this stage, the inside of the scope is pressurised using a pump with a pressure gauge (Figs. 8.5 and 8.6). This is to test for defects in the cover of the scope before any form of washing or immersion. One must ensure that the connection from the pressure gauge to the scope is secure, or leaks may arise from this point. Once this is done, pump the pressure up to that recommended by the manufacturer and observe the gauge for any drop in pressure over a couple of minutes, which would indicate a leak. Dry testing detect any large disruptions of the cover.

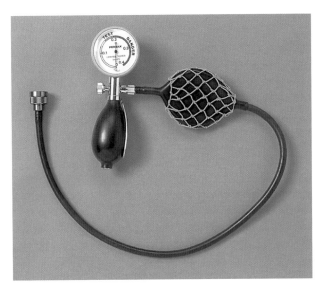

Fig. 8.5
Pressure gauge for leak testing. Note how the gauge has
markings indicating the correct working pressure.

Wet testing

Make sure that the ethylene oxide-venting cap is
not attached. Failure to do this can result in fluid
entering the scope. Attach the leakage tester prior to
immersion.

In this stage the test is performed as above, but
with the scope immersed (Fig. 8.7). If there is a
puncture in the outer cover of the scope a tiny
stream of bubbles will be seen emanating from
the defect. This test detects the smallest of leaks
and shows their position. Do not remove the
leakage tester until the scope is removed from the
fluid.

Some automatic sterilisation machines have a
leakage tester built in, but make sure that it operates
at the manufacturer's recommended pressure.

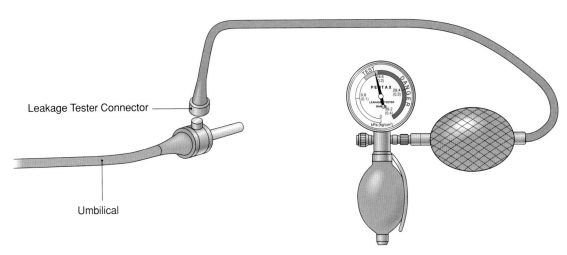

Fig. 8.6
The ethylene oxide connector point on the scope doubles up as the leak test connection point. This is on the umbilical of a normal
scope and on the control body of a portable.

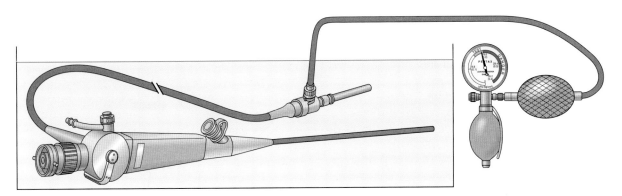

Fig. 8.7
Leak testing with the fibreoptic laryngoscope submerged.

Sterilisation/Disinfection

Chemical sterilisation

Most scopes can be sterilised by soaking the submersible parts of the fibreoptic laryngoscope in a chemical solution and by flushing the solution down the working channel. It is best to check with the manufacturer's recommendations concerning which solution should be used. Most advise using a fresh solution of 2% glutaraldehyde for 20 minutes, but 0.5% povidone iodine can be used. Any iodine must be wiped from the lenses of the scope as it can cause discoloration. It is best to avoid over treating the scope with any of these solutions because they can, with time, degrade the outer protective cover of the instrument.

Before immersing or flushing through the working channel, ensure that the ethylene oxide cap has been removed (if not, fluid will enter the scope and ruin the fibreoptic bundles). Also, substitute a 'cleaning cap' for the suction control valve (with a portable scope, if the battery pack or umbilical is detached then another cleaning cap should be fitted.) These caps ensure that the irrigating fluid passes down the full length of the working channel (Fig. 8.8).

Following sterilisation, wash the scope with fresh water, flush out the working channel and rub 70% alcohol over the non-immersible sections of the instrument. The scope is then left to dry before being placed in storage for the next occasion. Be sure to dry the electrical contacts before putting the scope away.

Automated sterilisation machines can be used with a fully immersible type of scope; these not only sterilise the instrument, but also wash it afterwards. They usually run for 20 minutes, but 1 hour may be necessary if the scope has been used on an infected patient. The scope is immersed in a bath of sterilising solution and the suction nipple connected to the sterilising machine via a small plastic pipe, which flushes the working channel. The machine can then be run through its cycle (Fig. 8.9). Always check and follow the instructions of the manufacturer.

Ethylene oxide sterilisation

Some scopes can be sterilised using ethylene oxide gas. Before sterilisation, attach the ethylene oxide-venting cap to ensure that the pressure inside the fibreoptic scope remains at atmospheric. If this is not done, the pressure inside the scope can build up and rupture the flexible cover of the scope.

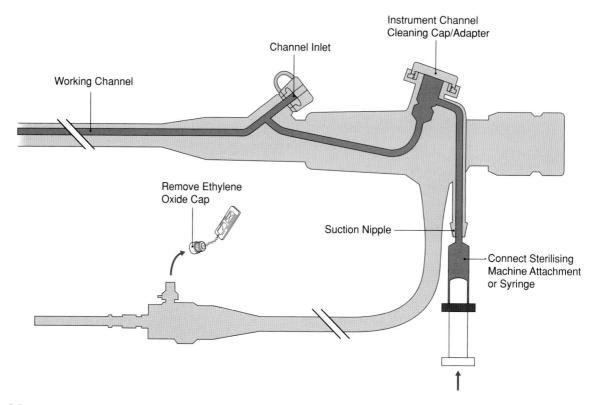

Fig. 8.8
Note the removal of the ethylene oxide cap and the addition of a cleaning cap where the suction control valve is usually situated.

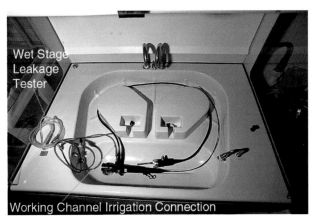

Fig. 8.9
Fibreoptic laryngoscope in an automated sterilisation machine. Note the green tubing connecting the sterilising fluid outlet to the nipple on the control body of the scope. On the far left is the tubing to connect to the scope to the leak tester.

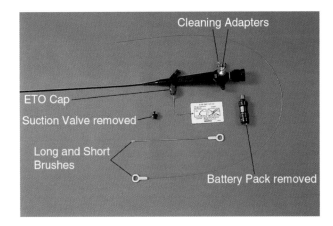

Fig. 8.10
Portable fibreoptic laryngoscope with its cleaning devices and the ethylene oxide cap attached directly to the control body.

To sterilise the fibreoptic laryngoscope, it needs to be subject to 10% ethylene oxide gas at 55°C (see glossary), under a pressure of 24 lb (see glossary) per square inch and a relative humidity (see glossary) of 50% for 4 hours (Figs 8.10 and 8.11).

Do nots

Do not rub any part of the scope vigorously or with any form of abrasive as it can damage both the

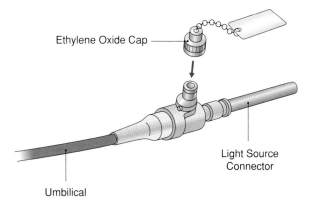

Fig. 8.11
Ethylene oxide cap attachment position on the umbilical.

lenses and outer protective cover of the instrument. Do not use boiling water or autoclave the fibreoptic laryngoscope.

SERVICING AND REPAIR

Servicing

There will be a servicing schedule recommended by the manufacturer and it is prudent to stick to it. If a scope is not serviced any warranty may be rendered null and void. Usually, manufacturers recommend servicing every 6 months and this should include a complete check of the instrument, cleaning of the working channel, adjustment of the tip angulation (the control wires stretch with time) and lubrication of the moving parts.

Repairs

Any part of the fibreoptic laryngoscope can be replaced, some parts being easier than others, and all but the simplest of repairs are expensive. The following are examples of approximate repair costs:

- Bending rubber (over tip) – approximate cost £250
- Whole insertion tube – £1700–2500
- Control wires – £750–1200

9

Teaching the technique

Learning fibreoptic intubation involves absorbing new information and concepts as well as acquiring visual-spatial and psychomotor skills. This is one of the reasons why the uptake and spread of the technique has been slower than would be expected. A failure to understand that it takes time to assimilate all that is needed to become proficient at fibreoptic intubation has led many people to try to perform this type of intubation without the necessary skills; failure and disillusionment coming close on the heels of their attempts. However, like many similar skills, with organised teaching and practice a high level of proficiency is quickly attainable. Attempts at real-life fibreoptic intubation then become highly successful.

If fibreoptic intubation is to become widespread, then it is essential that all anaesthetic departments have at least one consultant not only trained and proficient at fibreoptic intubation, but also involved in the dissemination of knowledge and skill to trainees. It has been suggested that every department should have an airway training room in which books, videos and CD-ROMs on airway management can be kept, as well as models and mannequins to practice on. As the airway expert, the anaesthetist has to learn and maintain his or her skills and to do so, facilities must be available.

SEE ONE, DO ONE TRAINING

The 'see one, do one' traditional form of teaching is one way to learn fibreoptic intubation. It has survived as the teaching method of choice in the medical world for hundreds of years. Most practitioners in the enlightened world of today will still have acquired their practical skills by this educational method. It is successful, but does subject the patient to the efforts of a complete novice and it assumes that the trainee has a good knowledge of the upper airway anatomy.

When learning how to perform fibreoptic intubation proficiently, it is difficult to assimilate the new information, the visual and motor tasks all at once. Therefore, if this is the technique by which the anaesthetist is going to learn fibreoptic intubation, at least 10–20 supervised intubations are required before an individual becomes proficient at the technique in the normal patient (some authorities recommend up to 40 intubations). Expertise will take a lot more regular practice. Those who have good visual-spatial perception and who are manually dextrous are more likely to succeed with this form of training.

In tandem with practical learning, the trainee must

also study the indications and techniques for awake and anaesthetised fibreoptic intubation, the various other techniques used to help with the technique, the problems encountered and how to solve them, and ethical considerations such as consent. The anaesthetist is also duty bound to ensure that when fibreoptic endoscopies are performed alone and on difficult airways, that they have a good array of airway skills as well as an escape plan for each intubation should anything go wrong.

GRADUATED TRAINING

In educational terms and with reference to the speed at which people become proficient at fibreoptic intubation, a graded or stepped training programme is hard to beat. In this system of training the technique is broken up into simpler sections so that the necessary skills can be acquired gradually, piece by piece, thereby building a solid technique. A graduated programme can be in the form of a course or workshop, or as part of an anaesthetic training scheme, in which case it can be performed more slowly. The minimum time needed to complete such a course is about 6–10 hours.

Example of a graduated training programme

Lecture(s)

In this introduction to fibreoptic intubation the following areas should be covered:

- Application of fibreoptic intubation
- The instrument and its care
- Local and general anaesthetic techniques
- Problems and how to overcome them
- Complications of the technique
- Some ideas concerning rescue plans

Demonstration of the fibreoptic laryngoscope

The instructor should demonstrate all the parts of the instrument, how to handle it and how to perform a fibreoptic endoscopy on a practice model, and finally demonstrate an intubation on a dummy or mannequin.

Practice on a model

Trainees should have one-to-one instruction, while practising on a model that teaches them how to manipulate the scope. These models are made as a

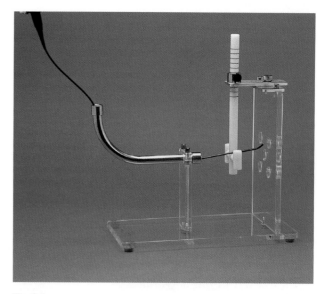

Fig. 9.1
Haridas–Hawkins fibreoptic practice model.

simple conduit through which the scope is passed and a target of holes in a backboard to aim at (Fig. 9.1). Initially, the trainee practices without looking through the eyepiece so that the results of each movement of the scope's controls can be seen. They then practice the same movements, while viewing through the eyepiece. Here trainees learn about the view obtained through a fibreoptic system, about image reversals and how to avoid the walls of the conduit, and how to aim the tip of the fibreoptic laryngoscope at the target.

Practice on a mannequin or live model

Again, there should be one-to-one instruction. The trainee performs an endoscopy on a mannequin and completes an intubation by railroading an endotracheal tube into the trachea of the dummy (Fig. 9.2). When a mannequin is being used, it is best to use a silicone lubricant regularly to prevent both damage to the scope and friction between the endotracheal tube and the airway. Some dummies are designed to allow the practice of a retrograde wire technique.

Some authorities use anaesthetised live pigs at this stage because the upper airway anatomy is similar to that of the human and the pig has few problems when anaesthetised.

Free practice

During this period, trainees can practice on any of the models and mannequins available and it is a time

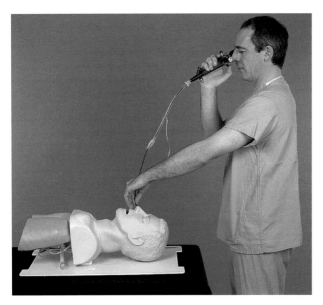

Fig. 9.2
A good scope position is one with a straight insertion tube and good control at the point where the insertion tube enters the dummy.

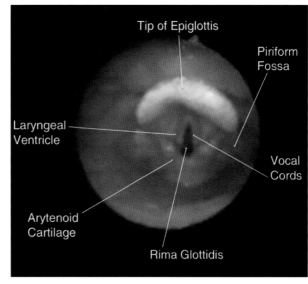

Fig. 9.3
A normal larynx as seen through the fibreoptic laryngoscope.

when particular points concerning the technique can be discussed with the instructors.

Practice of airway endoscopy

This is the first time that trainees are able to apply the skills that they have learnt, in a clinical setting. Some programmes have the trainees perform airway endoscopy as far as the larynx on each other after simple local anaesthesia. Patients undergoing or recovering from general anaesthesia can be utilised for the same purpose and endoscopy can be safely accomplished if performed when the endotracheal tube is still *in-situ*. Alternatively, trainees can visit the Ear, Nose and Throat clinic and use a nasendoscope, while some training schemes have included sessions in a bronchoscopy suite. This allows the trainee to become familiar with the problems of 'red out', secretions and upper airway movement. The trainee also comes to appreciate that the laryngeal view from the endoscope is different to that seen during a normal laryngoscopy (Fig. 9.3).

Practice of fibreoptic intubation on normal anatomy

Practice of fibreoptic intubation on normal anatomy can only be done in the theatre setting. Some authorities have used awake, sedated patients who require intubation for a surgical procedure, but the majority of trainers utilise patients under general anaesthesia. It is less stressful for the trainee if the patient is anaesthetised and avoids subjecting the patient to the discomfort of an awake procedure. A difficult airway can be mimicked in the normal anaesthetised patient by limiting any head, neck and jaw movements. According to General Medical Council guidelines, patients must give consent for these procedures because they are of an educational nature.

Free discussion

Here the trainees can ask any final questions and provide feedback to the instructors on their feelings about the content and presentation of the workshop. They can offer advice, either on the course or the technique itself. The trainees can also fill in audit forms so that the strengths and weaknesses of the teaching can be identified.

Difficult airway intubations

Difficult airway intubations can rarely be planned as part of a training scheme and so opportunities must be taken when they arise. The first few difficult airway intubation should be performed under instruction and can involve either a local or general anaesthetic technique.

The problem with workshops

Dedicated teaching courses or workshops can be expensive in terms of time and money, which tends to limit the number of practitioners who may benefit. Now that there are organised training schemes for anaesthesia in many countries, a useful addition to any scheme would be an 'airway' module during which graduated training in fibreoptic intubation can be accomplished.

TEACHING FIBREOPTIC INTUBATION UNDER GENERAL ANAESTHESIA

Initially, teaching on a patient who has received a muscle relaxant is useful, especially as the trainee is more likely to stimulate the larynx, trachea or carina accidentally with the scope. Following pre-oxygenation, 3 minutes is usually available in which to intubate the trachea before re-oxygenation is required. A total intravenous anaesthetic technique is particularly useful as it minimises the risk of awareness. Alternatively, intermittent positive pressure ventilation can be performed during the attempted intubation. This can be achieved using an oral airway with a chimney, or nasopharyngeal airway, which can be attached to the anaesthetic delivery system. However the rest of the mouth may need to be occluded with tape to allow adequate ventilation (Figs 9.4 and 9.5).

Others have used a Laryngeal Mask Airway, which is removed when the tip of the scope sits just above the mask. This method has the advantage that it minimises the duration of apnoea, but removal of

the mask must be done carefully to avoid damage to the tip of the scope (Fig. 9.6).

Training programmes in the past have used spontaneous breathing techniques. However, these are associated with a high incidence of coughing, laryngospasm and desaturation. However, the benefit of such a technique comes from having the airway moving in time with respiration, which mimics the awake situation.

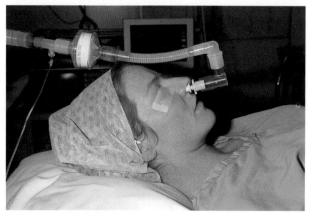

Fig. 9.5
A nasal airway is connected to the anaesthetic delivery system using an endotracheal connector pushed into the nasal airway.

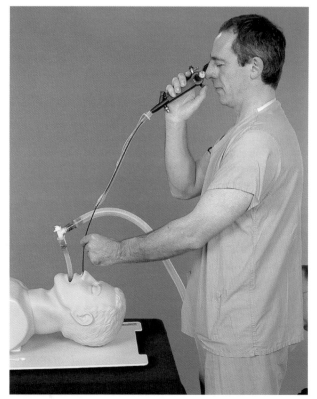

Fig. 9.6
The patient is kept anaesthetised and oxygenated via the laryngeal mask while the nasoendoscopy is performed.

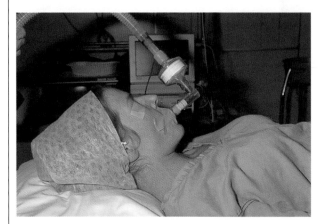

Fig. 9.4
A chimney oral airway is taped in to allow positive pressure ventilation.

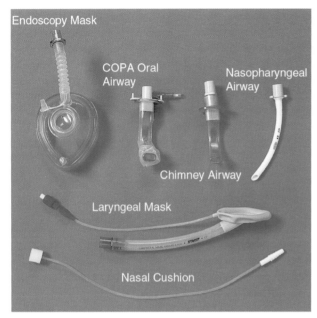

Fig. 9.7
Set of ventilation aids. The nasal cushion can supply
supplemental oxygen during an awake intubation.

An endoscopy mask can be used for patients
breathing spontaneously as well as those requiring
intermittent positive pressure ventilation. However,
it is wise to ensure that the endotracheal tube can
pass through the endoscopy diaphragm before
beginning (Fig. 9.7).

TEACHING AWAKE FIBREOPTIC INTUBATION

The technique of awake intubation should be taught
as part of every fibreoptic training scheme. The
knowledge needed to perform good local
anaesthesia, with or without sedation, can be taught
in the classroom. The difficulty comes in finding
cases to observe and later on to intubate. If there is
an airway training programme in a hospital, the
trainee(s) on that module can be called as a routine
when a difficult airway arises. Others have canvassed
patients to find individuals who are willing to
undergo awake, sedated intubation for their
operation, despite there being no need for the
patient to be awake. There is an ethical question
about whether this is right, as a significant
percentage will find the intubation unpleasant.

DUAL VIEWING

One of the problems encountered when teaching
fibreoptic intubation skills on a patient using a

normal fibreoptic laryngoscope is that only one
person can look through the eyepiece. Moving the
scope back and forth between trainee and instructor
not only takes time, but frequently it will be found
that the movement of the scope has altered the
view. This makes identification of anatomy and the
diagnosis of problems difficult. One way to avoid
this is to have a teaching side arm attached to the
fibreoptic laryngoscope to allow both instructor and
student to view simultaneously.

Beam splitting teaching attachment

This is a side arm attachment that fits over the
eyepiece of the scope and splits the light so that
~60% of it goes to the endoscopist and 40% is sent
down the sidearm to another eyepiece. This allows
both the trainee and the instructor to view at the
same time. The only problem with this system is that
the image brightness is degraded and consequently
these attachments are far less popular now that
video-teaching systems are available at a similar cost
(Fig. 9.8).

Video monitor viewing

Video camera attachments fit over the eyepiece of
the scope and transmit the image seen at the
eyepiece to a television monitor (Fig. 9.9). In this
situation neither trainee nor instructor can view

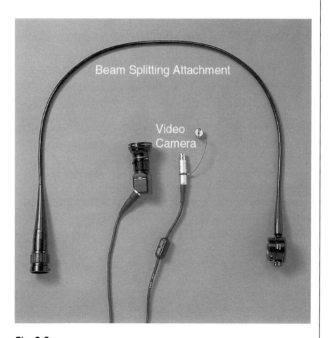

Fig. 9.8
Teaching attachments. The right hand arm of the video camera
plugs into the video control unit head (see glossary).

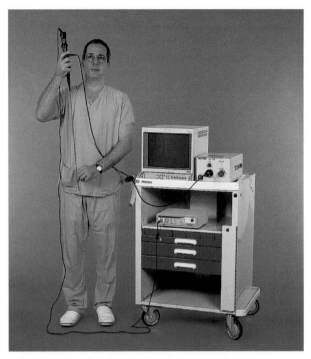

Fig. 9.9
A video camera-monitor system that can be plugged into a video recorder. The scope can be held as shown or the control body can be held over the shoulder.

through the eyepiece, but the monitor image is brighter and much larger than that seen through the eyepiece. An added advantage of this technique comes from the ability to videotape the fibreoptic intubation, which allows feedback when it is viewed later.

Before performing an endoscopy with a video camera system the 'white balance' button on the video capture unit must be pressed while the scope is pointing at a piece of white paper, to ensure that the colour balance of the image is accurate and life-like.

OBTAINING IMAGES FOR TEACHING PURPOSES

Still photography

By attaching a dedicated or modified single-lens reflex camera to the eyepiece of the scope it is possible to take photographs of the endoscopic view. The manufacturer can give advice about the best set-up for a particular scope and light source. With a xenon light source, a daylight-balanced 400 ASA film (see glossary) is appropriate, while a halogen light source requires tungsten-balanced film, rated at 320 ASA or above. However, these systems are less popular now that images can be taken from a video system and saved on a computer storage medium.

Videos

It is easy to obtain video footage of a fibreoptic intubation using a video camera attached via a video capture unit to the scope. A good audio-visual department can easily edit the film obtained and still images can be taken from any individual frame of the film at this stage.

Access to a computer with a video capture card (see glossary) allows digitisation of the video as 30–60-second clips, which can then be stored on the computer's hard drive or on a CD-ROM (see glossary). The more random access memory (RAM) available the better; 128 RAM is good and the faster the computer's processor (MHz) the better the quality of capture and playback. It should be remembered that an uncompressed capture of a 60-second clip can take up to 600 megabytes of disc space, but this can be compressed to just a few megabytes once it is on the hard drive. Video-editing software such as Adobe Premiere is required to do this.

Consent

When obtaining a permanent record involving a patient, informed consent should always be obtained, as detailed in the General Medical Council pamphlet *Making and Using Visual and Audio Recordings of Patients*.

REINFORCEMENT OF SKILLS

In many countries, the difficult airway requiring fibreoptic intubation does not appear on a frequent basis. It is therefore essential for all practitioners who have undergone basic fibreoptic intubation training to continue to practise their skills on normal patients during routine work.

APPENDIX

Bibliography

Bainton CR. New concepts in airway management. *Int Anesth Clin* 1994; 32, 4. Little, Brown and Company, Boston

Benumof J. Management of the difficult adult airway. *Anesthesiology* 1991; 75: 1087

Gillon R. *Principles of Health Care Ethics* ISBN-0471 93033 4 (John Wiley & Sons, 1994)

Hecht E. *Optics*, 3rd edn ISBN-0-201-30425-2 (Addison-Wesley, Longman, 1998)

Latto IP, Vaughan RS. *Difficulties in Tracheal Intubation*, 2nd edn ISBN 0-7020-2116-4 (W.B. Saunders Company Ltd, 1997)

Making and Using Visual and Audio Recordings of Patients (General Medical Council Publication, September 1997), 178 Great Portland Street, London W1N 6JE. Tel: 020 7915 3604 Fax: 020 7915 3558. Publications Tel: 020 7915 3507 Fax: 020 7915 3685 www.gmc-uk.org

Morris IR. Fibreoptic intubation. *Can J Anaesth* 1994; 41(10): 996–1008

Norton ML. *Atlas of the Difficult Airway: A Source Book*, 2nd edn ISBN 0815 164 335 (Mosby, 1996)

Ovassapian A. *Fiberoptic Endoscopy and the Difficult Airway*, 2nd edn ISBN 0-7817 0272-0 (Lippincott-Raven, 1996)

Randell T, Hakala P. Fibreoptic intubation and bronchofibreoscopy in anaesthesia and intensive care. *Acta Anaesthesiol Scand* 1995; 39: 3–16

The Report of the National Confidential Enquiry into Perioperative Deaths 1996/1997 (National Confidential Enquiry into Perioperative Deaths, 1998) ISBN: 0 9522 0695-1 Tel: 020 7831 6430 e-mail: info@ncepod.org.uk

Rushman GB, Davies NJH, Cashman JN. *Lees Synopsis of Anaesthesia*, 12th edn ISBN: 0 7506 3247-X (Oxford: Butterworth-Heinemann, 1999)

Seeking Patients' Consent: The Ethical Considerations (General Medical Council Publication, 1997), 178 Great Portland Street, London W1N 6JE. Tel: 020 7915 3604 Fax: 020 7915 3558. Publications Tel: 020 7915 3507 Fax: 020 7915 3685 www.gmc-uk.org

Shaw JD, Lancer JM. *A Colour Atlas of Fibreoptic Endoscopy of the Upper Respiratory Tract* ISBN: 0-8151-7720-8 (Wolfe Medical Publications Ltd 1987)

APPENDIX

II

Conditions associated with difficult intubation

Predictors of a difficult intubation

- Buck teeth or overgrowth of pre-maxilla
- Diminished atlanto-occipital joint movement
- Diminished mandibular protrusion (subluxation of temporomandibular joint)
- Increased alveolar–mental distance
- Increased posterior mandibular depth
- Laryngeal tilt
- Limited mouth opening – inter-incisor distance < 3 cm (see glossary)
- Mallampati score
- Obtuse posterior mandibular angle
- Receding mandible
- Sternomental distance < 12.5 cm
- Thyromental distance < 6–7 cm

Jaw problems

- Ankylosis of the temporomandibular joint
- Mandibular fractures, especially bilateral
- Mandibular hypoplasia
- Trismus

Neck problems

- Ankylosing spondylitis
- Burns or radiotherapy contractures
- Cervical instability – Down's syndrome, types of dwarfism and fractures
- Cystic hygroma
- Giant goitre or post-thyroidectomy bleeding
- Head halo
- Large abscesses
- Neck fusion
- Osteogenesis imperfecta
- Psoriatic arthropathy
- Rheumatoid neck
- Rigid neck collar
- Still's disease
- Vertebro-basilar insufficiency with neck extension

Oral problems

- High arched palate
- Induration of the floor of the mouth
- Lingual tonsil and Quinsy
- Macroglossia
- Micrognathia
- Prominent upper incisor teeth
- Submandibular masses

- Tonsilar hypertrophy
- Tumours

Facial problems

- Gross facial oedema or cellulitis
- Paget's disease
- Trauma

Pharyngeal problems

- Abscesses and oedema
- Ludwig's angina
- Sleep apnoea
- Supraglottic webs or mucosal folds
- Tumours

Laryngeal problems

- Anterior larynx
- Laryngeal deviation
- Laryngeal tumours/cysts

Tracheal problems

- Stenosis
- Tracheal deviation

Soft tissue trauma, swelling and scarring

- Angioneurotic oedema
- Burns and their scars
- Epiglottitis
- Epstein–Barr infection
- Facial cellulitis/oedema
- Facial trauma
- Laryngeal trauma
- Neck trauma
- Radiotherapy/surgical scarring

Syndromes

- Achondroplasia
- Anderson's
- Apert
- Beckwith–Wiedemann
- Binder
- Carpenter
- Chotsen

- Christ–Siemens–Touraine
- Cornelia de Lange
- Cowden
- Crouzon
- Cushing's
- Dandy–Walker
- DiGeorge
- Down's
- Ellis–van Creveld
- Engelmann
- Franceschetti–Zwahlen–Klein
- Freeman–Sheldon
- Goldenhar
- Goltz
- Gorlin–Chaudry–Moss
- Gorlin–Goltz
- Greig
- Gruher
- Hallermann–Streiff
- Hallervorden–Spatz
- Hanhart
- Hunter
- Kasabach–Merritt
- Kleeblattschädel anomaly
- Klippel–Feil
- Kocher–Debré–Sémélaigne
- Larsen
- Madelung
- Marfan
- Marie–Strümpell
- Meckel
- Melnick–Needles
- Millers
- Möbius
- Morquio–Ullrich
- Mucopolysaccharidoses – Hurler's/Hurler–Scheie
- Multiple epiphyseal dysplasia
- Nagars
- Noack
- Noonan
- Patau
- Pfeiffer
- Pierre Robin
- Pompe
- Pyle
- Rieger
- Saethre–Chotzen
- Schwartz–Jampel
- Seckel
- Silver–Russell
- Smith–Lemli–Opitz
- Soto
- Sprengel's deformity
- Stein–Leventhal
- Stickler
- Treacher–Collins

- Turner
- Ulrich–Feichtiger
- Urbach–Wiethe
- Von Recklinghausen
- Werdnig–Hoffmann
- Wolf

Others

- Acromegaly
- Morbid obesity
- Pregnancy
- Scleroderma

APPENDIX

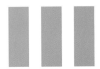

Facts and figures

(these are taken from the academic literature)

FAILURE RATES

All	1.2–1.6%
Accident and Emergency	13%
Railroading	1–2%
Nasal/LA	1.1% (n = 712) (see glossary)
Oral/GA	2.1% (n = 335)
Oral/LA	1.6% (n = 974)

DIFFICULTIES IN RAILROADING AN ENDOTRACHEAL TUBE

All	5–90% reported; expect ~25% but varies with technique
Nasal/LA	6% (n = 633)
Oral/GA	20–35%
Oral/LA	29% (n = 836)
Oral/GA/insertion tube	• 3.7 mm – 35% • 5 mm – 11%
With 90° anticlockwise twist of endotracheal tube	0–7%

Other complications

Coughing	16%
Difficulty in passing a nasal tube through the nose	26%
Epistaxis	8.2–22%
Fogging	18%
Gastric fluid in pharynx	0.05%
Hoarse voice	53% (n = 57) • mild – 44% • moderate – 7% • severe – 2%
Laryngospasm/LA	2.5%
Nasal mucosal dissection	
Oesophageal endoscopy	
Oesophageal intubation	9%
Pain/haematoma at cricothyroid stab	1.6%
Recall/LA/sedated/nasal	49%. Unpleasant in 8.7%. Of all patients, 1.5% said they would not like it again. The most vivid recollections were from those with little or no sedation due to the severity of airway compromise

Recall/LA/sedated/oral	40%, unpleasant in 5.1%
Retro-pharyngeal abscess	
Retro-pharyngeal dissection	
Secretions causing problems	22%
Soft tissue infection	
Sore nose	2%
Sore throat	39% (*n* = 57) ● mild – 28% ● moderate – 9% ● severe – 2%
Transient aphonia	< 2%
Vomiting/LA	< 0.5%

LOCAL ANAESTHETICS: MAXIMUM DOSES

- Lidocaine – 3 mg/kg (but more is safe in anaesthesia of the upper airway. Exact safe amount not determined.)
- Cocaine – 1.5 mg/kg (on nasal mucosa)

DISTANCES

- Nares to epiglottis – 15 cm
- Trachea – 10–12 cm, with 15–20 cartilaginous rings

WHAT FITS INTO WHAT

Laryngeal masks	LMA's will accept the following endotracheal tubes: ● size 3 = uncuffed 6 mm ● size 4 = cuffed 6 mm ● size 5 = 7 mm Intubating LMA = 8 mm
Endotracheal tubes	Those fitting into each other: ● uncuffed 5 mm into a 7 mm ● uncuffed 5.5 mm into an 8 mm Lubricate the inner well

FIBREOPTIC INTUBATION

	Endotracheal tubus Inner Diameter (ID mm)	Endoscope Outer Diameter Distal end (mm)	Endoscope Outer Diameter Inseration tube (mm)	Endoscope type
Adults	>7,5	5,9	6,0	FB-19TX FB-18X FB-18RX FB-18P FB-18BS
	6,0–7,5	4,8	4,9	FB-15X FB-15P FB-15BS
Children	4,0–4,5–5,5	4,1	4,2	FI-13P
		3,4	3,5	FB-10X FI-10P2 FI-10BS
Infants	3,0–3,5	2,4	2,4	FB-7P FI-7P FI-7BS
Premature infants	<3,0	2,4	2,4	FB-7P FI-7P FI-7BS

APPENDIX IV

Useful addresses

Cook (UK) Ltd [retrograde wire kit], Monroe House, Letchworth SG6 1LN, UK; tel.: 01462 473 100; fax.: 01462 473 190; www.cookgroup.com

Difficult Airway Society, c/o Dr Ian Calder, Honorary Secretary, Department of Anaesthesia, National Hospital for Neurosurgery, Queen Square, London WC1N 3BG, UK; tel.: 020 7829 8711; fax.: 020 7829 8734; e-mail: icalder@aol.com

Freelance Surgical Promotions [VBM fibreoptic intubating airways, endoscopy masks)], Unit 2, Olympia House, Beaconsfield Road, St George, Bristol BS5 8ER, UK; tel.: 0117 941 4147; fax.: 0117 941 4848; e-mail: sales@freelance-surgical.co.uk

Intavent Ltd [laryngeal masks and associated endotracheal tubes], Burney Court, Cordwallis Park, Maidenhead SL6 7BZ, UK; tel.: 01628 594 500; fax.: 01628 789 400

Pentax GMBH, Medical Division, Julius–Vosseler–Straße 104, 22527 Hamburg, Germany; tel: ++49 40-5 61 92 0; fax: ++49 40-5 60 42 13; www.pentax-endoscopy.com

Pentax UK, [fibreoptic laryngoscopes and related equipment] Pentax House, Heron Drive, Langley, Slough SL3 8PN, UK; tel.: 01753 792792; e-mail: info@medical.pentax.co.uk; www.pentax.co.uk

Sims Portex Ltd [exchange catheters/intubation guides], Hythe CT21 6JL, UK; tel.: 01303 260 551; fax.: 01303 266 761

INDEX

Sponsored by **PENTAX**

Pentax GMBH, Medical Division
Julius–Vosseler– Straße 104
22527 Hamburg, Germany
tel: ++49 40-5 61 92 0; fax: ++49 40-5 60 42 13
www.pentax-endoscopy.com

Pentax UK, [fibreoptic laryngoscopes and related equipment]
Pentax House
Heron Drive
Langley
Slough SL3 8PN, UK; tel.: 01753 792792
e-mail: info@medical.pentax.co.uk
www.pentax.co.uk